"But in the case of the smallest and the greatest happiness, it is always just one thing alone that makes happiness happiness: the ability to forget, or, expressed in more scholarly fashion, the capacity to feel ahistorically over the entire course of its duration. Anyone who cannot forget the past entirely and set himself down on the threshold of the moment, anyone who cannot stand, without dizziness or fear, on one single point like a victory goddess, will never know what happiness is; worse, he will never do anything that makes others happy."

—FRIEDRICH NIETZSCHE
UNFASHIONABLE OBSERVATIONS

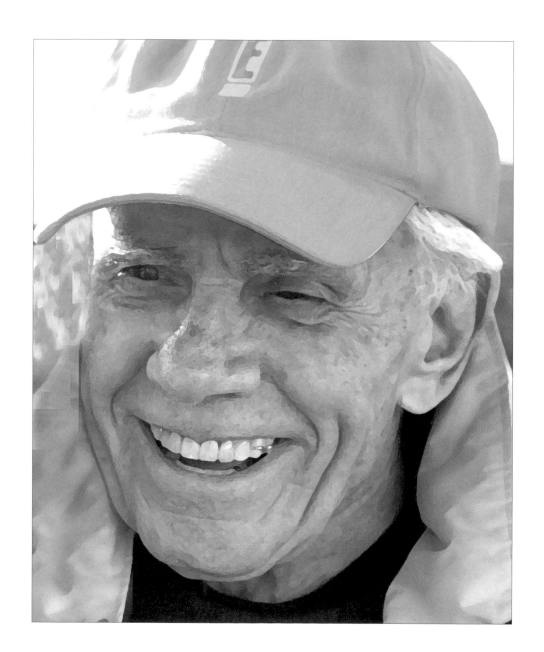

CONVERSATIONS WITH ED

Waiting for Forgetfulness: Why Are We So Afraid of Alzheimer's Disease?

ED VORIS

NADER SHABAHANGI

PATRICK FOX

IN COLLABORATION WITH SHARON MERCER

ELDERS ACADEMY PRESS
432 Ivy Street
San Francisco, California 94102
www.elderspress.org

ELDERS ACADEMY PRESS
432 Ivy Street
San Francisco, California 94102
www.elderspress.org

First Edition
Copyright ©2009 by Ed Voris, Nader Shabahangi, and Patrick Fox.

Cover + Interior Design: Tobie Smith Design
Production Design: Finley Kipp
Founding Publisher: Nader R. Shabahangi, Ph.D.
Managing Publisher: Elke Tekin
Photos courtesy of Ed Voris and Nader Shabahangi. Cover photo by Nader Shabahangi.

Elders Academy Press' publications are available through most bookstores. Substantial discounts on bulk quantities are available to corporations, professional associations, and other organizations. Email books@pacificinstitute.org for details and discount information.

ISBN 978-0-9816248-0-8 (Hard Cover) ISBN 978-0-9816248-1-5 (Soft Cover)

Library of Congress Cataloging-in-Publication Data
Voris, Ed.
 Conversations with Ed : waiting for forgetfulness : why are we so afraid of Alzheimer's disease? /
Ed Voris, Nader Shabahangi, Patrick Fox ; in collaboration with Sharon Mercer. -- 1st ed.
    p. cm.
 ISBN 978-0-9816248-0-8 -- ISBN 978-0-9816248-1-5
1. Alzheimer's disease--Popular works. I. Shabahangi, Nader Robert, 1957- II. Fox, Patrick. III. Title.
RC523.2.V67 2009
616.8'31--dc22
                    2009016744

Conversations with Ed is sponsored by **Pacific Institute** and the **AgeSong Senior Communities**, and published by **Elders Academy Press**, a program of **Pacific Institute**.

Pacific Institute is a nonprofit educational organization that promotes awareness in the way we understand aging, growing old and the role of eldership. It does so through two beautiful assisted living communities in San Francisco — Hayes Valley Care and Laguna Grove Care — as well as through counseling, education and publication.

Elders Academy Press seeks to change our view of aging from an undesirable process to an understanding of aging as important for our continued maturation in becoming elders. The Press thus seeks to encourage people to approach aging with appreciation and awareness so we might give back as elders to the generations that follow us.

To all caregivers who have placed their lives in the service and care of others: Thank you for continuing to be an inspiration for all of us.

TABLE OF CONTENTS

"I don't have extraordinary nerves or anything like that. I'm not any different than other people in that I get scared."

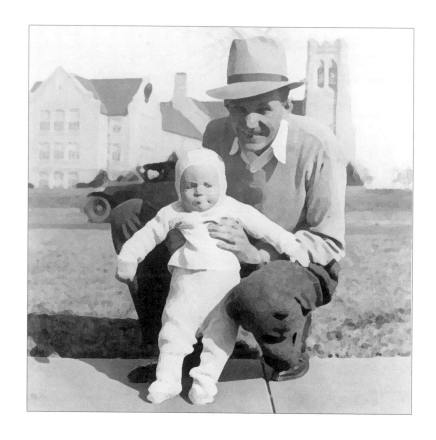

Conversations with Ed – BEGINNINGS

Pat Fox and I met for the first time at the University of California, San Francisco (UCSF). We were sitting around a table discussing ageism, issues of discrimination and diversity training, as well as general questions related to elder care. A few years later we had the idea that we should write something together on the attitudinal shift toward dementia, understanding it more as another state of consciousness and reality instead of labeling it as a disease. We began collaborating on an article that sought to identify the social forces at work in American society that create and sustain the predominately negative images of older adults who are forgetful, and to suggest that as a society we need to begin to explore the phenomenon of forgetfulness with greater openness. The goal of this endeavor was to promote the idea that there is much to learn from forgetful people if we are sensitive to what they offer us.

While still working on the article we met Ed Voris, a builder and retired sales executive who just a few months earlier had been officially diagnosed with dementia by a medical doctor in Southern California. Ed was interested in our approach to forgetfulness, because it was the first time that he had heard of someone speaking about all its possibilities.

Pat and I thought we should both meet with Ed and see what we could learn together. This was the basis on which we started our conversations with Ed.

Given our academic backgrounds, we had originally planned a more formal research project, but a more conversational format naturally developed which we videotaped. Thus, the present format of *Conversations with Ed* was born.

The meetings were initially intended to explore the phenomenon of forgetfulness and Alzheimer's disease from Ed's firsthand perspective. While we usually think of researching a topic of interest as requiring a rational approach or plan, we have consciously not traveled that path. This was liberating because of the radical openness to embrace the phenomenon of forgetfulness with no specific agenda or plan beyond learning. We agreed to let the interactions among us lead the way.

That is not to say that each of us came to the project as a tabula rasa, with a blank slate. Pat had been trained in psychology and sociology, Ed in theology and business, and I in literature and psychology. As with everyone, our respective formal training and life experience provide each of us with ways of ordering our perceived worlds – it cannot be otherwise. At the same time, by allowing the free play of our individual perspectives and biographical experiences, we created through our interactions something that is more than the sum of its parts. To those parts was added the skill of Sharon Mercer who was part of our meetings and edited the transcriptions. Her sense of narrative and enthusiasm for the project was essential to the creation of this book.

— Nader R. Shabahangi

THE EYE SEES ONLY WHAT THE MIND IS PREPARED TO COMPREHEND.

— *HENRI BERGSON*

THE VISION

The exploration begins as an initiation to a journey and leads to a vision of the possibilities of exploring forgetfulness as we age. We believe such a journey will ultimately yield an open horizon of meaning that has yet to be perceived in our society. Although we are aware that Alzheimer's disease has a host of diverse expressions, we emphasize forgetting as a central theme and refer to it as forgetfulness. "Dementia" literally means away from mind, and since we are still exploring what mind is, referring to someone as being away-from-mind makes little sense.

Some may be taken aback by the question posed in the book's subtitle: *Waiting for Forgetfulness: Why Are We So Afraid Of Alzheimer's Disease?* After all, how can we not be afraid of Alzheimer's disease? How can we not dread aging? By posing these questions we are inviting alternate ways of seeing Alzheimer's disease as well as aging. In so doing we do not want to minimize the suffering that people may experience watching a loved one become forgetful. Nor do we want to minimize that becoming forgetful and growing old can be painful processes.

What we are stating is that we have become socialized to believe that forgetfulness and aging can only be negative phenomena. Our society has a set of blinders on that negates our individual and collective ability to see the deeper meaning of what is called dementia and Alzheimer's disease and the deeper meaning behind the aging process. When there is a substantial disruption in our lives such as an unforeseen injury or illness, or the death of someone close to us, we apprehend meanings and possibilities that previously eluded us as we go about the routines of our everyday lives. Dementia is just such a disruption. Our aging process presents just such a possibility.

As the title of this book suggests, we have only begun to identify the meaningful possibilities of forgetfulness and aging and have chosen our words to highlight that potentiality. We hope to contribute to expanding the horizons of meaning associated with our conceptions of time and its fellow traveler, forgetfulness. This book wants to create a positive cultural space for people who have dementia and for those who accompany them on their journey. It is a book that we hope will alleviate much of the anxiety surrounding this phenomenon.

"I read in a book that 'with every loss of each brain cell, a part of the psyche disappears,' and then I wrote myself a note: 'But are we sure that's the truth?'"

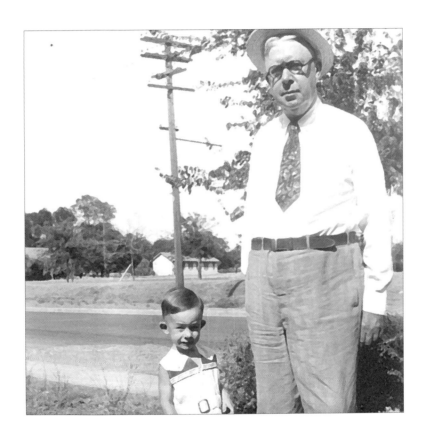

Introduction to
A Dark Night of the Soul

A man lies alone in his bed. A pressure lies like wet wool on his brain. It has been a tiring day, yet he sees no possibility of sleep. The only way to calm his spirit and find rest is to recite his mantra, one he has recited thousands of times.

Yet when he opens his mouth, no words come. Not a one. He knows that it is a simple mantra, but he doesn't remember it. Like the flavor of music heard from another room, he can pick up the rhythm of the mantra, but no words. None. It is the dark night of the soul.

Jumping out of bed, he pulls open dresser drawers, searching until he finds his mantra written on a piece of paper. Clutching the paper to him, he reads the words he used to know so well, "May I be filled with loving kindness. May I be well. May I be peaceful and at ease. May I be happy."

Meet Ed Voris. In the summer of 2007 Ed got a letter in the mail informing him he had dementia. That letter caused Ed to suffer. But then gradually a change took place in Ed. He grew excited about the opportunity his dementia had given him. Like a spelunker descending into the heart of the earth, Ed decided to explore the possibility that his suffering was attached to a certain way of who he was and what he was. Did he suffer because he was focusing on what wasn't? Or did he accept what was? Was the glass half empty or half full?

Each person we encounter provides us with an opportunity to grow in awareness, especially that person who challenges us. People can be at your side and face the journey of life with you or they can retreat. Facing the journey with someone who has been diagnosed with dementia is harder in some ways, because that person is going to have to face her fears, her anxieties, her own dark nights of the soul. But she is also going to share in your discoveries.

We believe it is important to be open to the gains instead of only the losses for people living with forgetfulness. Alzheimer's disease is one of the most feared symptoms we connect with aging. It is seen as a robber of people's minds, leaving them an empty shell. This is commonly accepted as truth, thereby diminishing the dignity of older people. But is there really nothing to gain from forgetfulness?

We started the conversations with Ed to explore this neglected side of forgetfulness and to search for its other meanings: What can it reveal about the deeper regions of our soul and our humanity? What can we gain through our encounter with forgetful people? What is it like to experience forgetfulness?

Together with Ed we decided to explore dementia from his firsthand perspective, and to see where that would lead us. The free play of our experiences and thoughts in the conversations showed the many facets of forgetfulness to us. We realized that if we anticipate only loss, enriching possibilities in our encounters with forgetful people would elude us.

As we discussed forgetfulness, we also dealt with issues surrounding our aging process. Many of us fear getting older. Here, too, it was important to shift our ideas of aging from a process of decline to a process of learning and *growing* old. Just as our mainstream value-set judges forgetfulness as a negative phenomenon, so it judges aging as an undesirable process often understood as a disease rather than an opportunity for growth.

Ed was our guide who made it possible to see the dawning of forgetfulness as an open horizon of possibilities and to look at aging with a fresh pair of eyes. We remember Ed saying repeatedly, "Use me, please use me in whatever way you can to further this worthwhile vision of yours." The degree to which we were successful in this endeavor is a judgment that only our readers can make.

"It's scary to think my brain might one day not even come up with one word to say."

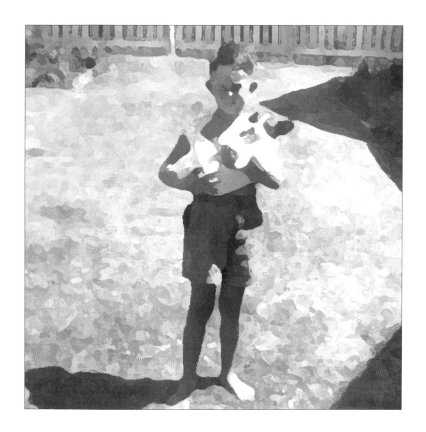

I CAN BELIEVE ANYTHING, PROVIDED THAT IT IS QUITE INCREDIBLE.

— *OSCAR WILDE*

THE INITIATION TO A JOURNEY

NADER: For me, the fundamental existential question remains: How do I choose to face what actually presents itself to me, especially if it challenges, pains me?

ED: There are two different stories that seem to me demonstrably true. One is that dementia or Alzheimer's is a terribly unforgiving and dreadful disease that seems to have one solution to all of this, and that is the end of life.

NADER: What is the other possibility?

ED: The other possibility is one that intrigues me. It's not as if I saw an open door and said, "Oh, boy. This is going to be good." It's scary to think my brain might one day not even come up with one word to say. But as far as I know, there is still communication even then. Communication with whom, what or how, I don't know. But hope has fueled my life.

NADER: So you can either look at it as a dreadful disease or you can look at it as an opportunity and a teacher. We tend to dislike a symptom because it's not what we are used to. However, in time we often come to understand that the symptom was a benefit for our life.

Like any word, *Alzheimer's* has multiple meanings. For example, a table can be something as simple as a makeshift table or something as grand as the banquet table in Versailles Palace. Some people have one image when you say *table*, and others have another image. Some people may not even know what a table is. So much of our understanding is contextually based.

ED: I read in a book that "with every loss of each brain cell, a part of the psyche disappears." And then I wrote myself a note, "But are we sure that's the truth?"

NADER: We are not sure. First of all, nobody has a clue what a *psyche* is. Second, "with each brain cell," that's an image as well. Is there really such a thing as a brain cell independent of my perception? Is it not what I impose on it? Don't we have an agreed-upon interpretation of what we see and then label it "brain cell?"

There is a famous story of Charles Darwin when he landed on an island and its inhabitants were wondering where he came from. And good old Charles is pointing to his boat, this humongous thing. And the natives keep looking, but they don't see it, because they don't have a concept of a boat. You and I would see a boat because we share a concept called boat, but for the natives, it was probably just a big, black blur.

ED: How do we create space for this mystery?

NADER: Is there a way we can get away from the sense of dread to a sense of: Wow, isn't it amazing what *is* now? Working with the cards that life deals you rather than wanting to have something else be there. That brings us to the question of what is good or bad about the loss of memory. And even this question is already problematic, that is directing what we encounter into categories of good and bad. How do we know what is good, what is bad? Our likes and dislikes, our preferences – from where do they come? On what are they based? No objective truth, no good and bad really exist independent of our judgment.

ED: For sure!

NADER: Forget for a moment the diagnosis of Alzheimer's and dementia, because in some ways they are just metaphors.

We do lose memory. The questions are: What are we losing and what do we gain? Am I locked into the idea that I need to remember your name in order to be somebody? Or, as was the case with some intelligence tests, that I need to know and remember a certain amount of words in order to be smart?

What other world are we slowly entering into with trepidation when we cannot reach any longer what we know? It's dark; it's unfamiliar. What are we entering into? Can we enter that world with curiosity rather than dread? Do we accept what *is* or do we suffer because we focus on what isn't? Ed, do you know the term *pathology*?

ED: Sure.

NADER: Today pathology means the study of diseases. But *pathos*, from the Greek, really meant suffering. So, pathology, the study of suffering, has turned into a study of diseases. Suffering has turned into a disease, something to be eliminated. Suffering is not seen any longer as an initiation to a journey.

ED: If you don't have the feedback from suffering, you have no way to improve your life.

NADER: Yes, and you don't have a motive to change. Dostoevsky was fond of saying that the origin of consciousness is suffering. In other words, there is little awareness without suffering.

We can also paraphrase Rilke and his lament that we humans are squandering our suffering. In my own experience, the suffering I experience is there because I am attached to a certain way of who I am and what I am, to a certain way of living my life.

So, in some ways you could say the moment you suffer you have been blessed, because you wake up from your attachments, from the routine way of living your life. The question then becomes: How can we conceptualize pathology as a journey into another world, into another reality that is not based on the way we customarily look at the world?

Ed: I have an eerie feeling when you say that, because I have been wrestling with that. I feel an excitement about the opportunity to explore the question. I use the term spelunking – going deep under mountains – which scares the hell out of me but I do want to. I don't have extraordinary nerves or anything like that. I'm not any different than other people in that I get scared.

Nader: We all have our own journeys of suffering and some of those have to do with our expectations, beliefs, wishes, and desires. Rather than seeing a beautiful sunny day out there, we mope and say, "Why me and how come?" We beat ourselves up for beating ourselves up.

I want to let you know that I'm not a stranger to suffering in the sense of the sleeplessness and the pain that comes with that. I feel that we can go through this together knowing that there is someone else who can say, "Hey, I'll be there with you, so you're not alone."

Ed: Like the magician who told his wife that he would come back after his death. They agreed on a date each year when he would come back to establish that he was still there, she just couldn't see him anymore.

I thought of that story with regard to my friends. My friend Bob has been a continual support. What Bob brings to my life now is his belief that my life has value, that I've done things that are meaningful to him. Therefore, I am alive. And so I realize I will not die alone.

A friend of mine asked me to be part of his burial team when he died. He made a do-it-yourself casket and he assembled all the parts. He had it set up so when he died his brother-in-law put the pieces together in a casket. And then his wife filled the casket with flowers so there were gorgeous blossoms cascading out of it. The six of us carried his body out and put him in the casket. Then we took the pre-built top and each of us screwed a screw in. The next morning the brother-in-law and his now widow drove him to the undertaker where he was cremated. But looking back and seeing him in that bed of flowers, the bed that is normally seen as a coffin...

NADER: ...made all the difference.

ED: Yes.

NADER: I've been thinking about your friend, Bob, and how each person we encounter gives us an opportunity to grow in awareness, especially those who are challenging us. I can either stand by your side and face the journey with you, or I can retreat. One most certainly is harder, because I'm going to have to face your fears, anxieties and pain together with you. And in doing so I will have to feel all of my own emotions as well and sometimes even more than you do, because we all have different sensibilities.

ED: Bringing confidence to each other by sharing, so we can both become bigger.

NADER: That's right. How, for example, can we see forgetfulness as something we don't understand yet? There is a Taoist story of a king who was hunting with his best buddy. The king goes to shoot an animal and somehow the gun goes sideways and the king shoots off his own thumb. He gets so upset that he says to his buddy, "How can you give me a gun that is not working properly?" and puts him in prison. A year later the king is hunting again and gets caught by cannibals who are ready to put him on the stake to eat him up. Just before they put him on the fire, they realize he has a defect in that he has a thumb missing and they can't accept that, so they release the king.

The king is now full of remorse, because he recognizes that if he hadn't shot off his thumb, he would be dead now. So he goes to his friend and says, "I'm sorry for putting you in jail." And his friend says, "I'm not sorry at all. I'm so happy you did." And the king asks, "How is that?" His friend says, "Well, in all likelihood I would have been hunting with you, and they certainly would have eaten me up because I am pretty perfect."

So from a longer perspective, it turned out to be a blessing, but at the time it was hard to think there was anything positive in it.

Ed: So how many times do you think we should meet like this? How long do you expect this to go on? Until I . . .

Nader: Until death.

Ed: I was going to say until I go into the rabbit hole.

Nader: Until we're going to put those screws into that bed of yours.

ED: That would work for me.

NADER: We are privileged to be on this journey with you, wherever it is going. I'll be frank with you. I have many ideas, and I have many strong convictions about being right, of course. And I have to say that these convictions are mostly based on my basic intuitive understanding of the world. So when you come along and you actually speak to it, it is a whole other level of acceptance or validation.

ED: This is a very exciting time for me. But I'm not going in the rabbit hole real soon.

NADER: I was thinking of that in terms of final years because neither you nor I know when our final days are going to be. I may be in that rabbit hole sooner than you.

ED: You remind me of a story I used to hear back home about the preacher who was sitting in his office and saw some kids in the church school playing and he decided to go out and interview them and see how church school was working in their life. So he looked at the first boy and said, "Do you want to go to heaven?" And the boy said, "Oh, no, Sir." To the second one he said, "Do you want to go to heaven?" and he said, "Oh, no, Sir. No, Sir." And the preacher looked down at them in exasperation and said, "You don't want to go to heaven when you die?" And the boys said, 'Oh, yes, Sir. Yes, Sir. We thought you were getting a load to go right now."

And so began the journey.

*"If you don't have the feedback from suffering,
you have no way to improve your life."*

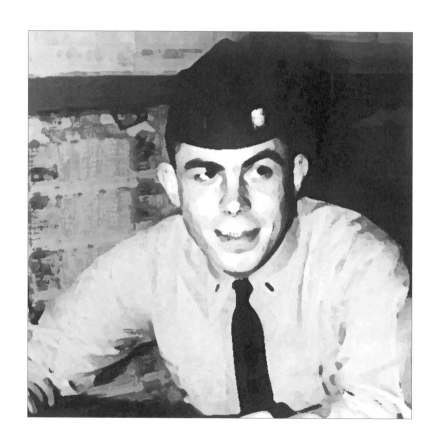

Chapter 2

THE GREATEST DISCOVERY OF MY GENERATION IS THAT A HUMAN BEING
CAN ALTER HIS LIFE BY ALTERING HIS ATTITUDES.

— *WILLIAM JAMES*

HOPE AS VERB

ED: As it does for many human beings, the concept of death invokes both anxiety and resolve in me. Anxiety because death is the ultimate unknown, resolve because finitude can be the greatest benefactor of the life we lead on Earth.

Steve Jobs, of Apple computer and a cancer survivor, put it succinctly in a graduation speech given at Stanford University: "No one wants to die. Even people who want to go to heaven don't want to die to go there, and yet death is the destination we all share. No one has ever escaped and this is as it should be, because death is very likely the single best invention of life."

I've been experiencing that personally. For me, it is like being born again into life in a new and refreshing and meaningful way. Whereas society and many of my friends view so-called old age as a place of dying, for me it's a place of living, a place of new invention, new challenges, and new hope as much as any other experience I've had in life, and more than most.

So I'm excited. When I was told last year that I had dementia, I had no idea what this meant for my life, because all I got was a little piece of paper from my doctor advising me that I had been diagnosed as having dementia. What does that mean? There was no one to talk to me about it or answer questions. All I got was a three-page blurb they sent me in the mail that told me to go pick up my new prescription. I had no idea what this Alzheimer's medication was. The only thing I knew to do was to see where this is going and find out what I can do about it and what I can learn and to act as responsibly for myself as possible.

So it's been a whirlwind for me and I suppose in some sense for you, because last year I had no idea who you were and now I feel a closeness with you that I feel with few people, and so we go on. I see this as an opportunity to bring some meaning to my life in these months or years.

PAT: What strikes me most is that there can be alternative scenarios for someone who is experiencing memory loss. Instead of demonizing it and classifying it as a disease, you can say what you are saying: that this is an opportunity for you to explore areas of your life that you might not otherwise have felt compelled to explore.

You were saying how the diagnosis gave you a different perspective on your life and your view toward death and the future. And I'm wondering if in our everyday lives when we're doing the everyday things we do, whether we get into a mode where everything is routine and we won't think about things other than the little pathways that are well worn in our behavior. And maybe sometimes it takes something like a shock to rattle one out of everyday existence to bring a new or different perspective on life and what you need to do with your life from now on.

That's an interesting avenue to explore as an alternative vision to your standard medical diagnosis. Rather than making it a disease and saying, "Well, Ed, he's got Alzheimer's. Stiff upper lip," which is the social disenfranchisement or pathology model, versus one where there is more of an integrative approach to it. So countering our commonly agreed upon reality, what Nader refers to as "consensus reality," is challenging. Your sharing of perspectives with us provides an outline of another way of living through dementia. But this means also thinking about Alzheimer's from the larger perspective of society and raising questions about how we think of memory loss in the context of everyday life.

ED: My ex-wife's father, whom I dearly loved, had Parkinson's. She was unable to go visit him or to bring him up to our house, because it depressed her so that she could hardly function. The result was that I went to see him. We'd talk and he was demented in a lot of his thoughts.

The only thing he wanted to talk to me about was when he was going to get his new car. And while he was talking about getting his new car, I was asking him how he was going to get his license renewed. He would be sitting there strapped into a wheelchair with a football helmet on his head so that if he fell over he would not bang his head. But he would talk to me with deepest urgency that he needed to get a new car.

For a while, I wrestled with that and kept trying to talk reason with him. Then, in a sudden bolt of lightning, I realized I didn't have to talk him out of it. He knew he couldn't have a car, but he needed the hope of selecting a car. So we would talk about cars that he might be interested in buying and how he was going to pay for one and so forth. He got a lot of emotional relief from talking about cars, and I didn't have to worry about him getting in his car and driving somewhere.

PAT: Your story points out something really important. I read an article that looked at cancer patients, their discourse around hope and how they conceived of hope. The medical folks use hope as a noun: "There is no hope. You are at term and there is nothing more I can do." And then there is hope as a verb when a person says, "I hope I can do this. I hope that this happens."

The way we talk is so important in terms of the concept of giving hope. It's not an unrealistic hope of some pie-in-the sky thing that is in reality never going to happen. It's a much smaller kind of hope. A hope of action. A hope of agency where people can get a sense they are still in control. There is a hope that they can do something about whatever it is. It gets back to what you were saying earlier about what does the word mean?

ED: That's because of the reputation of Alzheimer's. Most people say, "You don't have Alzheimer's." The way I speak I guess I'm more articulate than a lot of people. But if you hear me try to describe some things you will notice that I've lost a lot of my vocabulary or the access to it.

PAT: I think that those reactions on the part of others are derived from this demonization of the disease. It's ironic in that in medicine they are striving to identify the so-called preclinical indicators of Alzheimer's under the assumption that medications introduced earlier in the disease process might have a more beneficial effect.

What that has done socially is create a space for people like you who have the label but are still able to interact in normal ways with people. And then people say, "You can't have Alzheimer's," because it doesn't fit their perception of a person sitting over in the corner staring off into space.

I don't think Nader and I would deny that there's something going on, especially when you yourself report that, "I can't remember things. I can't find words. I can't put my sentences together." There's obviously some kind of change that you're experiencing. But I think our point is to try to get the larger society to understand that there is variation. That just because you have the label doesn't mean one thing. It means many different things.

It's made worse when you get a label like Alzheimer's where you are totally disenfranchised, because nobody thinks you can be human or you can communicate. That's our interest in being with you on this journey, to see from a firsthand perspective.

Ed: A lot of it has to do with helping people learn how to take care of one another. And the individual is not given a whole lot of attention, because we don't have a public relations agent going to the Congress and the Senate and universities and so forth.

Pat: That's an interesting observation, because what that may require is to not make Alzheimer's a disease to the extent that we, as a society, have done. It would probably allow for alternative visions of the meaning of the disease to arise such as those we have been discussing.

Ed: You don't have to pathologize it in order to say it's doing something and let's find out what it is.

Pat: But up to this point in time, by and large it's been demonized by the advocates as part of what one observer has called the "health politics of anguish" in the United States. The way our political system is structured, you have to show how bad something is in order for the public to get behind it and for Congress to get behind it. Alzheimer's is just one disease in a long string of diseases where that has happened.

Ed: But when I went to the Alzheimer's Association wanting to participate they asked, "Where is your advocate?"

Pat: Your caregiver?

Ed: Right. They wouldn't talk to me.

PAT: That is a concrete example of the disenfranchisement of the person with Alzheimer's disease, because the focus has been on how to support the caregivers. This is, of course, not a bad thing. But the primary emphasis has been on getting funding for biomedical research and second on care. And even in the care realm the historical focus has been on the caregiver, not the person with Alzheimer's disease.

But what they're having to deal with now, Ed, is people like you who get diagnosed early and can talk about their experience and can say, "Wait a minute. I'm still here. I'm still a human being who has feelings and thoughts." They have to take that into account now.

ED: They don't want to.

PAT: They have been thinking that way for 30 years. It's a hard thing to shift overnight.

ED: Well, I hope they do it soon.

"Whereas society and many of my friends view so-called old age as a place of dying, for me it's a place of living, a place of new invention, new challenges, and new hope..."

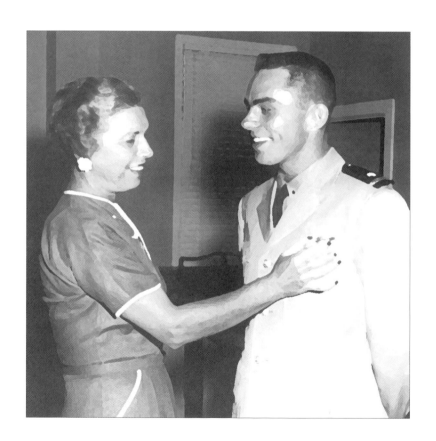

Chapter 3

THE MOST BEAUTIFUL THING WE CAN EXERIENCE IS THE MYSTERIOUS.

IT IS THE SOURCE OF ALL TRUE ART AND SCIENCE.

— *ALBERT EINSTEIN*

A HAPPINESS ALSO FALLS

NADER: There is an eloquent expression by the German poet Rainer Maria Rilke. He writes: "And we, who think of happiness as climbing, feel the emotion which almost overwhelms us, when a happiness falls." What does that mean? Well, normally we see happiness as a movement that lifts us higher, often in terms of receiving more earthly possessions, more in terms of meeting our expectations of living a so-called good life. But happiness can also show itself through what we might at first understand as a tragedy, as an unwelcomed event. It is just these events, however, that push us to deepen who we are, deepen our understanding of life, of mystery.

Take another poignant statement by Rilke: "Dare to say what you mean by apple." Dare to say what you mean by what you have just summarized with this quick little five-letter word: apple. If we didn't have the word apple, what would you call it? What is this thing that evokes memories, taste, smells, and texture and all kinds of mythological meanings?

What do we mean by dementia, Alzheimer's, cancer, any of those diagnosed disease-labels that often obscure the richness and mystery of the meaning that lies behind these conditions?

Pat: In a sense it is a byproduct of the use of language, like that beautiful quote about the apple. Apple is a word we use to communicate for practical purposes. So you can say, "Okay. Pat brought an apple to eat."

Ed: Is it a Golden Delicious?

Pat: Somebody might ask that, but in everyday life, we are generally on to other things and we're not involved in trying to understand the immediacy of the phenomenon. We are more interested in what are we going to do next. I think the medical construct of Alzheimer's disease and forgetfulness associated with it is something we take for granted in our society. This can result in not even entertaining the idea that there may be other ways of seeing the phenomenon because we tend to accept medical expertise and the visions of forgetfulness that arise from it.

It is interesting what you are saying, Ed, in terms of being a person who wants to live his life a certain way: "Yes, I have this dementia. It is classified as a disease, but I don't want to go down that path." It takes somebody with a hell of a lot of guts to not be forced down that path by the most well-meaning relatives, health professionals, and others. As a society we do not allow people to do that.

NADER: I think of the quantum view of the universe in which we each create our own reality in a constant feedback loop with what we encounter outside of us. Actually, the quantum view challenges the very existence of categories such as inside and outside. We influence what we see; what we see influences us. The way I look at the world determines how I want to see life and my role in it. We can understand our lives as case histories, a compilation of data and facts as is done in medicine and the social sciences: "You are this age, that tall, this heavy. These are your blood samples and values, and this is your medical history and your genealogical predispositions, and so forth."

We can also look at our lives as soul-stories, as lives that have purpose and meaning. From the point of view of soul-stories, we see what happens to us as purposeful, not accidental or random.

The question becomes: What is the soul wanting to figure out? How does the soul want us to live? Seen within such a context, the events in our life become fascinating encounters for the soul to work through. Chronic illness and other symptoms are then expressions of the soul wanting to communicate, wanting to express itself through you. Remember that the Greek word *sumptoma*, at its most basic meaning, meant that something "befell" you. The word *symptom* does not imply that something is good or bad, just that something happened to you. How we see what befalls us is up to us: do we see it as a teacher, or do we categorize it into something good or bad? To see what befalls you as teaching you something is a much richer and, so I feel, more rewarding view of life.

Ed: Let's say we are social revolutionaries and we have a plan with regard to the nature of life as we encounter it. We undertake a plan to spread vital, meaningful life to 100 years of age, and we have a program designed to begin working with that right away. I don't know how we'd do that. I'm just saying it excites me to think about this.

Until she died, my mother was terrified of death. She did not want to talk about it, because it terrified her so. My sister died at 49, my father at 60, so the landscape, as I saw it, was relatively limited; you can't farm beyond here because your plants will die and you'll die with them. Then suddenly the barn door flies open and I can see the possibilities of life as far as the hills.

They tell me that someday I will have lost my language. I don't know what I'll do then, but it's not true now and there is no reason I have to quit now.

I'm more excited than my younger friends who are 50 and even some of my friends under 50. I'm excited and I don't know of anything that brings more meaning to life than to have someone around who is excited.

When I retired at 65, I decided to go to Washington to live on retirement and be near my son and daughter-in-law and grandkids. I hadn't been there much more than a year, when it was discovered I had major obstructions in all four valves in my heart. So I had a quadruple bypass, which was not a very pleasant experience. I had some problems. Anyway, the ultimate thing is, in case I didn't tell you, I lived.

Pat: I was waiting for that. Thanks for clarifying that.

Ed: After the quadruple bypass, I started to look at what to do. I decided to work with developmentally disabled people. What a fantastic time that was in my life. I taught them how to cook, helped them with their jobs, and got tickets to go to a baseball game. My life had so much meaning then. It was rich.

Pat: The example that you gave for working with developmentally disabled people reminded me of one of the most satisfying jobs I've ever had, when I worked as an activity director in a nursing home. My job was to show movies, play bingo, and try to engage the folks who lived there in things that they found interesting.

It wasn't complicated or hard work, but it was satisfying in the sense that you felt you made a difference in these people's lives, because most of them didn't have any connections to the outside world. Some did, but most didn't. So, even the smallest things people were excited about and looked forward to doing.

It's an interesting fact that many of the things that are the most meaningful are the ones that are less valued from the standpoint of the overarching economy and status systems of the society. Caregiving is an example of that.

Ed: No one ever became a millionaire taking care of developmentally disabled people. I've had a lot of friends who've made considerable wealth and I've never known any of them who were made happier and enjoyed life more. They became more aggressive and more separating rather than joining and sharing. Far from experiencing a time of fear and doubt, I feel privileged to be able to use my life to possibly make a contribution. No money – just life – used for all of us. Can it get better than that?

PAT: It goes back to what Nader was saying earlier about the quantum universe and living in a world that has meaning.

One example of that is the idea of earlier times where death was seen as a mystery. The death of a person was seen as a sign of some greater power, which came and took the person away. Over time, especially in Western societies, we've reduced that mystery to the body. "What's wrong with the body and how can we do something to the body?" In the meantime, we've lost the context of meaning of that larger power that in the past we surrendered to.

NADER: I was reading a wonderful poem by Mary Oliver yesterday. There is one line toward the end, "When death comes, I don't want to sigh or be frightened or have that feeling that I've simply visited this earth. I want to have lived it."

So if we weren't to call it Alzheimer's disease that you are living, Ed, what would we call it? What happiness befell you? What are you lucky to have been burdened with, so to speak? Can we live in these questions?

PAT: Can we tolerate the ambiguity?

"Far from experiencing a time of fear and doubt, I feel priviledged to be able to use my life, possibly make a con-tribution. No money – just life – used for all of us. Could it get better than that?"

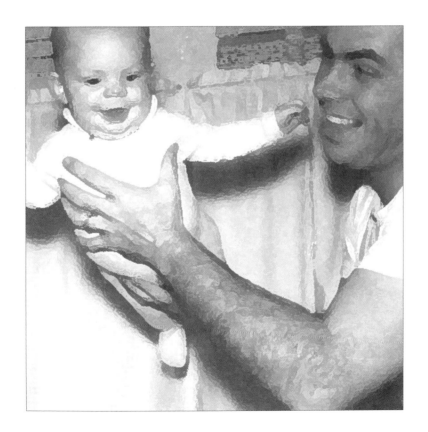

Chapter 4

THERE ARE NO FACTS, ONLY INTERPRETATIONS.

— *FRIEDRICH NIETZSCHE*

WHAT IF ALZHEIMER'S WAS REDEFINED AS SAINTLINESS?

ED: I genuinely feel privileged to be chosen to have dementia, if that's what I have. I may just be crazy; maybe you can be both. Anyway, I am having the time of my life. I feel that part of what I have for myself is to make the most of the opportunity.

I don't want to be an alarmist saying, "I did this, and it had to be Alzheimer's." It could be old age. It could be a cold or a virus. I don't know how to characterize whatever is going on in my body, except to say I do feel change almost like a tide. There is something around memory loss and my waking up in the middle of the night and not being able to finish the words. That happened last night, and it is becoming recurrent. It seems as if what I'm doing is pushing back the tide and someday it will slip over.

PAT: When you mentioned you would wake up, was it that you would wake up from a dream and try to remember the dream?

ED: No. What I've been talking about is my mantra. It is something I'm intimately familiar with and I use it every day, but in the middle of the night I can't call it back. Or I can call back part of it and part of it I can't. By persistently working with it for two, three, four, five or six times, it comes back fully.

There are some things about my language in this. I wasn't even aware of all the elements of language until I did this, but there is the lyrical part, there is the simple language part, and the way the rhythm builds. So I could say, "May I be filled with loving kindness." I usually don't have a problem with the first part, but "loving kindness" is not language that I customarily use in my life. So I'll stumble over that. Sometimes I'll have the rhythm but not the words. "May I be filled with duh, duh, duh, duh . . . ."

I never had a problem with this before, so I am getting an experience with Alzheimer's itself. We're looking at each other over the trench and I'm saying, "You better dig in because I'm not letting you through here." But it just laughs and says, "You dumb shit. In six months you won't know loving kindness from jack."

PAT: So you are aware that you're having difficulty finding words.

ED: I am learning there are a lot of things that are going on, that have begun to develop, that I think may be a bad habit of upsetting moments because of Alzheimer's. For example, last Friday I somehow walked away from my suitcase at the airport. And my suitcase didn't have the good taste to follow me. It stayed right where it was. Fortunately, they had it in Security and when I went back there on Tuesday, I was able to recapture it.

PAT: Looking back before you were diagnosed, can you remember if something jogged you to think something like Alzheimer's might be happening?

ED: I was getting really concerned, because Alzheimer's doesn't introduce itself and say, "If you don't mind, we're going to come in and work on your brain for a while." There was no notice that someone moved into my body and was doing things, so there was no way to understand. I noted a number of things that happened and I didn't know then and I don't have any proof now that they happened because of Alzheimer's. I just know that a whole number of incidents took place.

The principal thing I was aware of was my vocabulary. It began as words and advanced or regressed to the point where I found myself beginning to have problems with sentences and structured thought. It starts off being separate words, and then they start to line up into paragraphs.

I may be erroneous in that this may have nothing to do with Alzheimer's, but these things had never happened before and they began to occur with increasing force.

One of the interesting things is I've lost a lot of the mental faculties that come to play in reading, so my mental skills slowed down. I keep reading the same chapter in a book three or four times, trying to go forward.

And I completely lost the ability to read in public. I'm in a meditation group and we frequently read things for group consumption, everyone reading in the circle. I had to stop, because I would read a line and I would start off fine, then I would slow down before I got to the end of the line and I couldn't continue.

And the incident I just mentioned, at the airport, the loss of things. I've never been a flake. Like everyone, I've lost things. I think everyone's lost a car in the parking lot once or twice, but I started doing it every week. I've spent countless times trying to figure out where my car is. Always before, I had some inner sense that would tell me, "You're in A14," or wherever, and I could walk over to A14 and there was my car. Now I have no memory of where I should look. And I should have made a note of it but I forgot. Or maybe I did make a note of it, but I lost it.

This is when I first learned of Alzheimer's and dementia, and the nature of it. I received this letter after never having a conversation...

Pat: With your physician?

Ed: Never a word.

Pat: Your physician examined you and then you got this in the mail?

Ed: Correct. It's a three-page letter that says "dementia," with care instructions.

Pat: When you got this in the mail, what did you think?

ED: What in the hell is this? I had requested three previous interviews to talk about my vocabulary, because I was having an increasing difficulty in explaining and describing things. I had one of those vocabulary tests, and I slid back severely.

PAT: What was the test?

ED: They give you ten words, and you have to repeat them back in order. I can't remember exactly, but things like that and other questions. I had been through this before.

PAT: So the sliding back was from your performance of the first time. What kind of realization was that?

ED: No one ever talked to me about it. I talked to myself, and said, "That's a bunch of crap," although I knew I had not done well.

The truth also was that I had two car wrecks in little over a year; the second wreck was a total. The other driver suggested that I somehow had some fault in it, which I knew, but I wrote a long letter about how the other guy did run into me, I didn't run into him. Afterwards, I knew that no matter who was at fault I was in trouble as a driver and that I had difficulty maintaining attention.

PAT: What was it that led you to that realization, since you were in denial mode up to that point?

ED: An abnormal day.

PAT: So you had a real bad day?

ED: For one day I was honest with myself. Everything was bad, honestly.

PAT: Was it a realization that maybe something was wrong?

ED: Something was wrong, yes.

PAT: The first thing you recognized was the inability to find words?

ED: Yes, my ability to remember and find words was always there before.

PAT: So, you would be communicating with someone and you would want to think of a word to communicate an idea, and you just couldn't find the word?

ED: Increasingly, I was stumbling in my conversation.

PAT: When you were doing that, what were the reactions of the people you were talking with?

ED: They tried to cover for me. People are pretty nice to you. Someone would say, "You know you are not able to articulate the way you used to." But getting the attention around this issue has not been as forthcoming as one could have wished. I did realize that things were sliding for a long time. I had to push to get attention for the problems.

PAT: I want to go back to your tests. Can you remember the first time you were tested by a neuropsychologist, and what that experience was like?

ED: It was boring, no challenge. I knew it 100 percent, and that's like saying

I'm one of the best students in my grade school at age 47. It wasn't any big deal, but there were memory challenges. This was short-term memory, of course. He'd read a number of words and then I would be challenged to quote them back and in order. That was a little more challenging but it wasn't any problem. But that last test, I really blew it. I couldn't remember.

PAT: What was the time from the first test to the last one?

ED: Two years.

PAT: Did you remember if they were doing the same test as they did the first time?

ED: It was similar in structure, but there was a precipitous drop in my score. Let's say, if you got everything right you got a 20 and I had about a 14, so it was substantial. It was beyond the normal range.

NADER: Has the test been repeated?

ED: Not since then, no.

PAT: Sounds to me like a mental status examination. See if this sounds familiar. What building are we in right now?

ED: Oh, yes.

PAT: Spell *world* backwards.

ED: Right.

PAT: Did you draw intersecting lines?

ED: I didn't do the pentagons, but I do remember having to interpret time and day and all of those things.

PAT: Exactly.

NADER: This reminds me of the inclusion of "spiritual emergence" as a relatively new diagnosis in psychiatry.

ED: Really?

NADER: Yes. I love that, because I remember reading the *Confessions* of Saint Augustine and how he describes his conversion to Christianity. Before this new diagnosis, modern psychiatry would say he had a psychotic break and major hallucinations, and this guy would have been pumped up on who knows what, perhaps even been locked up for awhile.

So you understand the power of a label: it can imprison you, it can free you.

So what is the test saying, really? Biological or neurological changes must parallel psychological and spiritual changes. You said you did lousy on the test you took. What does that mean? Your test results actually showed some kind of a transformation that was going on with you, no? So what if I interpret your results differently? What if I saw Alzheimer's as a symptom of spiritual emergence? What if I redefined Alzheimer's as saintliness?

ED: Then I would definitely be an Alzheimer's patient.

"I've had a lot of friends who've made considerable wealth and I've never known any of them who were made happier and enjoyed life more."

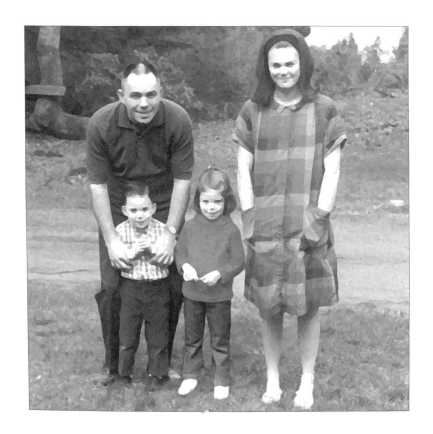

WHAT'S IN A NAME?

ED: The way I saw the test was that there were simple challenges I couldn't do. It didn't measure the outer reality, just my ability to use mechanical equipment to tell me whether it was three or nine o'clock.

NADER: For me, I was thinking about how I don't care so much about doing something in the way I used to.

ED: I've changed in that way, too.

NADER: Working with people who are forgetful has helped me to become more accepting of my own changes in priorities as I age. I used to get upset if I didn't remember a phone number. Now I don't, because I don't think it is so important to remember everyone's phone number. I am becoming more accepting of who I am and what *is*. So it's a different focus.

ED: I've been involved in church and politics, so I went to a lot of meetings where I'd meet a number of people. There's a certain benefit to being able to say, "Pat, where's your friend, Nader?" Most memory work has to do with social occasions rather than with a cold, statistical test.

PAT: There was a sociolinguist who did a study of one person whom she interviewed over the course of Alzheimer's. And the point you're making, Ed, is a key point she made after writing about 200 pages. She observed that those types of artificial situations are not good measures of the capability of someone to interact with people in social contexts, as opposed to a contrived clinical context. The tests that you were taking are part of this reductionistic model that decontextualizes individual experience and instead tends to focus on specific aspects of cognitive functioning as measured on a standardized test. "OK, we are now in the parietal occipital lobe and that's where we are going to test your ability."

The kind of process you went through decontextualizes the person as a social being and places him or her in a clinical setting that is controlled by a system of thought.

NADER: I'm noticing, as we're talking, that we are focusing so much on memory, which is already part of the paradigm, because everybody has told us Alzheimer's is about memory loss. What I'm saying is that we are already in that box and it's about memory, but what about other things that happen? What about a person becoming more quiet, gentler, or more forceful? Or more present and more loving with what is? We don't even look at those variables and categories of change.

PAT: That's important, because the biomedical model is one that is being spread worldwide and it attempts to counter some of these alternative ways of thinking or seeing forgetfulness.

NADER: That's right.

PAT: There is this wonderful book that's called *No Aging in India*. Lawrence Cohen, an anthropologist from Berkeley, wrote it. One of the points he makes is there is no Alzheimer's in India, because they interpret the phenomenon and its symptoms as a problem with the family.

This is ironic, because in the United States in the 1950s some psychiatrists conceived of senile dementia as sociogenic. The idea was that the reason people start to forget, withdraw, and show the symptoms of dementia, which at that time was seen to affect men more than women, was that men's social roles upon retirement were drastically changed. Men all of a sudden went from defining themselves as the contractor, the builder, or the executive to retirement. And when you take those roles away with retirement, as well as the lessening of income and other kinds of status, people withdrew. It was seen that it didn't affect women as much because they were at home, fulfilling their expected social roles, and they could still do so.

NADER: There's something you mentioned, Ed, that intrigues me. You said it is helpful in certain social settings to remember people's names. So much depends on, "How are you doing, Jim? How is your wife,

Anne?" That is what makes that connection and it's good for business.

ED: If you're selling, you know, if you can start off by saying, "Hi, Jim. Good to see you again. How's your wife, Anne?," you are halfway to an order.

PAT: I guess that's why I was never a salesman.

NADER: Me neither. This is why I found what Ed was saying so surprising.

PAT: I think that's because I never conceived of myself as somebody who was good at that. There is something about interacting with people whom you haven't met before. I don't know what it is, maybe it's just nervousness or it's a new experience.

But I'm concentrating on being nice to somebody I've just met. So I say, "How are you doing?" and shake their hand. And the person is telling me their name, and it's just gone. Then I go, "Oh my God! I just met this person, and I can't call him Ed or Schmed because I don't remember his name!" Then you think you remember it, but you say, "I can't say it, because what if I'm wrong? I'm going to look like an idiot."

ED: If you talk to people about it they will say, "We're all that way." That's why I go back before I leave and say, "You know what? I've forgotten your name. Can I get it again, because I was really pleased to meet you?" The important thing is to get an affirmative connection before you let it go. Then you greatly improve your chances of remembering the name.

PAT: It's an embarrassing example of the world you worked in that required that. And that it was a very important thing you had to do in order to make these connections.

NADER: That's right. That's why I was so surprised when you made it instrumental. I never think of it that way, because I have the luxury not to need to use that skill.

ED: The most beautiful sound in the world is the sound of my own name.

NADER: Is that right?

ED: Everybody's is. No matter how shy or withdrawn they appear, there's nothing they'd rather do than be remembered by somebody.

PAT: I don't know about that. I don't think I'm that way.

NADER: Me neither.

PAT: Maybe it's because my name is Patrick. I went to Catholic school, so you'd think that Patrick would be a great name to have, but it was something that never sat right.

ED: Mostly every March.

PAT: Yes, around the 17th, when you drink green beer. But I always wanted to not be in the line of fire and I don't know why that is.

ED: I'm sure you're pleased when someone notices you.

PAT: Yes, the recognition of others is important. That's absolutely correct.

ED: It's also good to have good feelings between people.

PAT: That's the important thing, because we see ourselves in the other in some way but not necessarily in a conscious way. When we see a person, we see fragments of who they really are. We probably never know who they really are, but those fragments are all that we have.

It's interesting, because the more you interact with someone, of course, the more fragments you can get. You get a fuller picture but not a complete picture. And the name is such an important thing to give them the notoriety of being an individual and not just one of the mass of people who are out there in the world.

ED: Then if you add the defining elements you have a choice. "I remember you. You're a fat person, right?" Now that is a really warm way to start a relationship.

NADER: I remember that in some forms of meditation there is an emphasis on going beyond likes and dislikes, beyond "I like this, I don't like that."

To prefer one thing to another is a recipe for creating unnecessary suffering. All kinds of absurdities can happen because of that preference.

I assume you are partly in a field, Ed, where you have moved beyond preferencing whether you remember something or not. Sometimes I ask a student, "Can you think of a part of your mind that would benefit from being demented?" Almost always, students can find that part. For example, they would answer that they would like their inner critic to be less vocal, would love their inner taskmaster, the one who doesn't want you to sleep late, the one with the never ending "to do" lists, to be more quiet.

When I wake up in the morning I normally follow up on something I did yesterday in the workday world. What if I could start fresh every morning? How much of who I am in the morning is dependent on what I know about myself from yesterday? And how much does my name say about my identity, really?

"If you could sell Alzheimer's to lonely people as a cure-all, you could get rich."

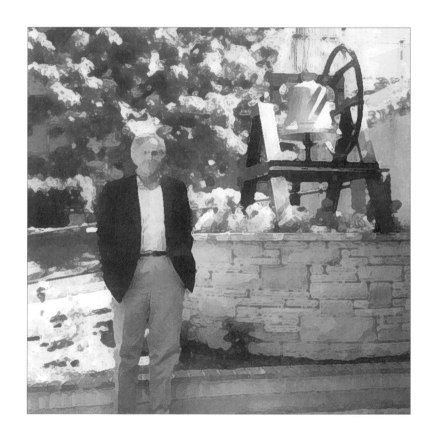

Chapter 6

LOVE CONSISTS IN THIS, THAT TWO SOLITUDES PROTECT AND TOUCH AND GREET EACH OTHER.

— *RAINER MARIA RILKE*

ALZHEIMER'S – A CURE FOR LONELINESS

PAT: In the context of the medical model, in what ways do you think seeing your physician and then learning you have Alzheimer's was beneficial for you? Or was it not beneficial for you?

ED: I could have looked it up in the encyclopedia. It didn't deal with me as a human being. It dealt with me as a piece of flesh, and flesh needs three of these medications a day, and two of these, and one of this. Alzheimer's was treated just like my cardiac bypass. It wasn't treated as if there was any beneficial thing I could take, although they did give me medications, which have profoundly improved my ability in all the areas we talked about.

PAT: For example, you could remember words more easily?

ED: All of those things I've mentioned are better. I have had fewer parking lot problems. I completely eliminated parking lot problems in October, when I gave my car to my daughter.

PAT: That's a big help. No car, you don't have to worry about getting lost in parking lots. So when you started taking the medication, how long did it take before you noticed a difference?

ED: It was probably two weeks, and then there was a growing awareness that things were pasted back together somehow. I have a lot of good day/ bad days. Things will be good for a day and then they are not so good, but for the most part it's much more up than it was.

The first six months of this year before the diagnosis were pretty rough, because I didn't know what was going on. I had problems on the job. I hired a woman to do the bookkeeping, because I couldn't keep up. That's where I assumed some sort of related connection to whatever was happening. I just couldn't produce. My mind was slow. I made notes each day. "Today I had a hard time doing this and that." I didn't know why I was experiencing these things.

NADER: I am curious about the response of others to you when you told them of your diagnosis. What were the reactions that you can recall?

ED: When my life was falling apart last summer, my son cared enough about me to come and help me move in with him. My kids, my friends, countless people reached out to me not to say, "Gee. I'm sorry you've got Alzheimer's," but just, "We really love you." They have been very caring. My friends have extended themselves in so many ways.

If you could sell Alzheimer's to lonely people as a cure-all, you would get rich, because everybody dies, but to die knowing you're loved and having that reaffirmed by your friends and others is so deeply meaningful to me, it is impossible to adequately describe.

PAT: So would you characterize those types of changes in your relationships with people that are important to you as a positive aspect of Alzheimer's?

ED: Immensely so.

PAT: Deriving from the diagnosis?

ED: Sure. The first step that really got people's attention, including my own, was the seriousness when I quit driving. They didn't say, "Ed, quit driving," they said, "Ed's unable to continue driving, so let's see what we can do to help him."

PAT: It is unusual that you decided on your own not to drive, because a lot of times people go into denial, like you described earlier. People do that, and families do that. A lot of times folks have to hide the keys or take the distributor cap off, because the person who has been diagnosed with Alzheimer's doesn't want to give up driving.

I was wondering in the process of coming to that decision, was it the accidents that brought that to your mind? It gets back to the question that you didn't really consciously know when that denial turned over to, if not acceptance, at least to an understanding of a different phase in your life as a result of Alzheimer's.

ED: It was a gradual process of changing. It was not an instantaneous thing. Then I said, "I've got to quit driving." I had two wrecks in the last two years, and it's a miracle no one was injured or killed in the second one, because it totally destroyed the car.

I reluctantly and fearfully gave up my car to my daughter, trying to lighten the load so I could focus on the most important things. And immediately I felt claustrophobic, because I was living with my son. He lives in a nice area, but there isn't any public transportation for a mile and a half and there are rough hills to walk. I thought I would blow my brains out the first two or three days.

PAT: Why was that?

ED: I was cut off from everything in my life. I could breathe. I could eat. I could take the dog for walks. But everything else I knew about life, like if I wanted to go to a movie, I couldn't drive there. I really felt just despondent.

Then various friends of mine said, "We will pick you up and take you. What do you need to do?" I participate in a meditation group on Sunday morning, and they set up a routine where somebody picks me up, and somebody takes me back, and we often have lunch.

So everything I thought I needed to get around was taken away from me, but it was given to me in another form that's just as effective and in many ways much more.

Nader: Why is that?

Ed: Because when I was driving in my car I was alone. I was lonely and separated, even though I had good air conditioning. So in many ways, my life is richer, because I don't have a car.

There are more people in my life. And not driving a car gives me a picture of a world that I didn't see when I was driving. Each day when I walk, I see and hear all the birds and animals that I didn't see and hear before. I don't think it is misleading to say I'm unquestionably happier and fuller with less.

The response of my friends has just been overwhelming. It's been so generous and caring. You could almost use that to talk people into getting rid of their cars and bumming rides.

I have been a fund-raiser for 20 years, and the most remarkable thing to me is that I discovered that people really need and want to make gifts. They want to help. Often they don't know how, but when they have an opportunity to help by giving a car ride, it makes their day. I think that awareness needs to be shared by more people. People need to understand that the best thing you can do for yourself is to give something to someone else. And it's not the quantity of the gift; it's the quality of the giving.

"I don't think it is misleading to say I'm unquestionably happier and fuller with less."

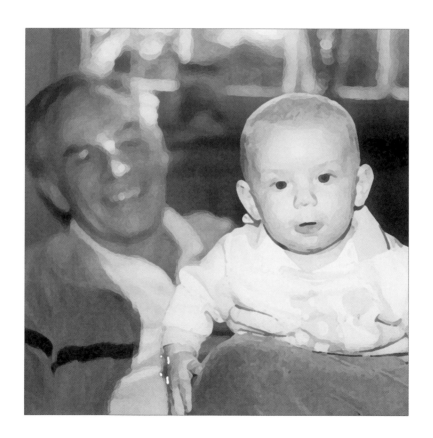

Chapter 7

EVERYTHING YOU CAN IMAGINE IS REAL.

— PABLO PICASSO

LET THAT REALITY GUIDE YOU

ED: One thing I wanted to mention to you is that I have seven years of graduate theological education, and spirituality has been central to my life. I think of it as around the corner and down the corridor. It's exciting to me to think of the possibility.

NADER: Spirituality is a bias we have in that we believe there is meaning to be found in whatever happens to us. How does that resonate when I say that?

ED: That's something I feel comfortable with, because I use it as a working hypothesis of life. I'm a recovering alcoholic. Next Thursday, I'll celebrate 22 years of recovery. My life has changed dramatically, not just from the ravages of alcoholism but also from the ability to focus more clearly in living my life around the concept of spirit.

PAT: Are some of the spiritual things inserted into some of the symptoms that are happening to you? As you were saying earlier, is there some kind of meaning that needs to be discovered, or is discoverable?

ED: It's difficult to attribute proof to it, but that doesn't mean that it's not true.

PAT: In one undergraduate course in psychology, there was a course on personality. The instructor assigned two books. One was about astrology, and the other was a standard psychology textbook about personalities. And everybody was making it a contest. Which source of knowledge was real, or more real?

ED: I've treated life pretty much like a visit to Disneyland; I've done what I was interested in, not worrying much about money. It's not as though I can get along without money, but it solves itself if I work and make a contribution. And that's what I have done. I've raised a lot of money and been involved in politics.

NADER: I like your treating life like a visit to Disneyland.

ED: It brings a certain amount of unreality to it, though.

NADER: I believe that those people whom we call exceptional mostly have had a somewhat different view and understanding of reality. We might even say that the source of creativity lies in our very ability to move away from the normative view of reality. Otherwise, how could we create anything new?

ED: As a matter of fact, there have been times when I didn't do anything. I gave away everything I had and put a $10 bill in the back of my wallet as my security. Then I did pickup work, as it came to me.

NADER: So in your present life, how important is your past to who you are now?

ED: I was an out-of-control drunk until I was 51. Twenty-two years ago, I woke up and said to myself, "You can't get away with this crap anymore." I joined Alcoholics Anonymous to get some structure to my life and begin to piece it back together.

In Alcoholics Anonymous there is a saying, "Turn your life over to your higher power, and let that reality guide you." That is very much like what you were saying about how you shape your own reality. But I don't feel I can do it independent of some higher power or sense of reality.

NADER: Remember that alcohol is also referred to as spirits. One might look at the person drinking alcohol as someone who is in search of spirit. The alcoholic is a person on a spiritual journey.

PAT: Like any other mind-altering drug, it is a way to get out of everyday reality. It provides you with a different way of seeing the world.

ED: I spent a lot of my life angry.

NADER: Angry at what?

ED: Life.

NADER: Why?

ED: I don't know. I just know that in the meditation, reading, and prayer I do as a daily exercise, I began to submit my life to other influences of love and forgiveness. Then a few years ago, I woke up one morning and I thought, "Something strange is going on. What on earth could this be?" Then I realized it was that I was happy. I was happy to start each day with the promise of being happy and wanting to contribute that. That was really magnificent.

Recovery from running away from your life with alcohol is not something where you say, "I gave up drinking and I'm okay," because I started at 14 and I really screwed up my life.

NADER: What do you think the drinking served?

ED: It was a screen to shelter me from the real challenges of life. I think in some ways I felt inadequate. Both my parents were alcoholics. I never had just one drink. It was like the hole I'd drop into to disappear.

NADER: So it would influence your whole day?

ED: And my nights and my relationships. It was the concept of running away from things.

NADER: There is one question that comes to me. You speak about being a recovering alcoholic and how you got in the Alcoholics Anonymous program, and how giving over to a higher power was part of the 12-step program?

ED: That is correct.

NADER: Do you feel the kind of practice you've had with those 12 steps made it easier for you to say, "It is time to stop. It is time to quit driving my car"?

ED: I never thought about that. My initial response would be to say absolutely, because Alcoholics Anonymous was key to my decision to turn my life over to the care of a higher power. And if you don't do that, then you haven't recovered.

NADER: You also mentioned something about your needs, that you found it amazing how your friends reached out to you after you told them about your diagnosis of dementia. Is that also a learning you received from Alcoholics Anonymous, to express your needs?

ED: It is certainly consistent with it. There is a process of having a sponsor who works with you to examine your life. You learn that recovery is learning to help other people take the steps that you took in your own life, and to support them in carrying those steps out.

PAT: Ed, you've talked about your experience with people who are in recovery. Have you ever had the opportunity to talk with other people who have been diagnosed with Alzheimer's?

ED: The Alzheimer's Association recruited a couple of guys who were in recovery. But there was not much talk with people with Alzheimer's. There were people talking about people with Alzheimer's.

PAT: I see.

ED: The first thing I did after I learned I had Alzheimer's was I said, "I don't know much about it, but I want to look into it and see what I can do to take care of myself."

So I called the Alzheimer's Association and this nice lady explained to me that they would be happy to assist me, if I would just identify the family member who was going to come with me. I said, "The person who is taking care of me is me." And she said, "We require that you have a family member attend with you." It's not like I was going to strip my clothes off, or do anything crazy. I was just trying to deal with Alzheimer's by myself.

PAT: This may be difficult to answer, but what are some of the meanings you have constructed around having forgetfulness and having Alzheimer's? Are you trying to find meaning in it?

ED: I got books to give me some insight into it, but there is a strange transposition. Is this true, or is this true? How can this be true, if this is true? Or are they both true?

PAT: One of the things is the perspective that has been created around Alzheimer's disease and caregivers. Lots of people do have Alzheimer's, but there has been very little voice from them until recently. The voices that have come out are the ones of the extremely negative seventh level of hell perception, which is caregivers seeing family members change in dramatic ways; when you're talking to them, they're not the person they used to be.

I was wondering whether you have had a frightening discussion about having Alzheimer's with your friends. We've talked about how some people have drawn closer and those have become more satisfying relationships. But have you had problems with the opposite? Were there any other reactions you can recall?

ED: I don't want to talk about it.

PAT: That you didn't want to talk about it or that they didn't want to talk about it?

ED: That they didn't want to talk about it. Oh, there were some long impassioned things like, "Sorry to hear that. It gets passed on down the road." I felt like they were uncomfortable with me. I felt they were doing things that they would just as soon not pursue any further in that there are a lot of choices in your companions, so drop this one.

A real question in my mind is why my lady friend of the last four years has been pulling back. There could be a thousand reasons.

I would just as soon not talk about separation from my lady friend. Let's talk about Alzheimer's and forgetfulness and dying.

"I've treated life pretty much like a visit to Disneyland; I've done what I was interested in, not worrying much about money."

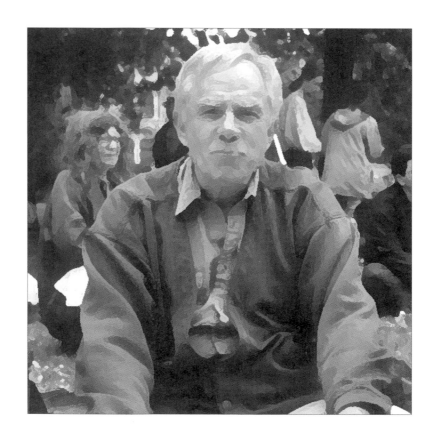

Chapter 8

Only those who attempt the absurd will achieve the impossible. I think it's in my basement — let me go upstairs and check.

— *M.C. Escher*

What if those Black Holes Were Gifts From The Gods?

(Pat was absent in this meeting, held up by an unexpected university faculty meeting.)

Ed: One of the issues I would like to raise is the moral career that commences upon the receipt of a medical diagnosis. I have had substantive changes occur in my life, because I have to accommodate these new things that enter into it, and I didn't even know what Alzheimer's was. So is it possible to talk about healing someone with Alzheimer's in connection with treatment?

Nader: We also have to ask ourselves what do we mean by treatment, because who is treating whom? We have an established power structure that is saying, "We know what is normal, and we will put our tools to work and treat you so you will be normal again." Someone who states that they can treat you, states that they know how to do something to you.

ED: And I don't know how.

NADER: And you don't know how. That's right. You are not being asked as if your own thoughts and ideas do not count. I think your earlier question is exactly that question of, "What is it?" How can you talk about something like Alzheimer's or dementia without having a clear understanding of what a mind is?

Before you talk about having "no mind," what do you mean by mind? The definition of a healthy brain based on a brain scan of an 18-year-old is based on biology only. What if that 18-year-old was someone who was emotionally withdrawn from others? Do we take that into consideration? So someone might biologically be considered normal or healthy, but from another point of view, be considered quite abnormal. Compare this to a brain scan of someone who is supposed to have a disease but who really sits quietly and acts gently with the world and himself. How do we define health and illness?

ED: Those are the things that intrigue me as a person with dementia. At least that's what I've been told. I've chosen so far not to have them saw the top of my head off to look and see.

But how can we discuss this in terms of where we are as a society and where are we going with it? And what are our hopes that we hold out to the people saying, "We can't promise you anything?" But we can say that these are the kinds of things we hope for, so that you can live with hope. And we can work together jointly to try and confront these things.

Another thing I would hope is that we could begin to understand elderhood as an integral part of our society. To know that elderhood is not a temporary holding spot until there's a plot in the graveyard.

NADER: The amazing aspect of elderhood — or old age as a phase in its own right — is how we apply different standards to it.

I was speaking to an elderly woman who said she didn't want to wear a hearing aid. It occurred to me that perhaps she no longer wanted to fit into the standard environment where speaking and hearing are important, that her reluctance to wear a hearing aid had to do with her need to pay attention to her inner voice. Maybe we need to teach others that there are ways of communicating that are beyond words, ways that are perhaps much deeper, much richer than the spoken word.

ED: Is the deterioration of memory a dream or is it reality? What is the loss of memory?

NADER: What is mind? What is intelligence?

ED: Is it the sense of what causes our emotionality, the cause of our self-interest? Suppose my mind became so still that even the sense of I was gone? Then there would be nothing that was apprehended. There would be no color, no shape of any kind, yet there would be clarity. There would be no grasping after I and mine, just a brilliant clarity. There would be total freedom in this clear, empty, unimpeded cognition.

NADER: There is a wide spectrum between normative science and mysticism. Then there is poetry, literature, and other creative modes of expression such as painting and music. There are all these different ways of looking at life.

But it seems we have become dominated by the modern scientific method having a stronghold on what is called truth. So we feel ashamed if we use other modes of seeing the world as an explanatory model. We often hear, "This is my feeling, but I have no scientific evidence," as if scientific evidence was needed to validate our feelings.

So in some ways we deny our intuition, our instincts, and our feelings. We deny our learning in other modes of perceiving the world by stating, "I need to take a look at what the scientists say about that." As if repeatability, measurability, and quantifiability – the hallmarks of the scientific method – were the way to see the world. Science, from *scientia*, really just means knowledge. And knowledge ought not necessarily be judged by how we obtain it. But the scientific method, Nietzsche once exclaimed, won out over science itself. Knowledge was only true knowledge if it was obtained via the scientific method.

That is part of the legacy of the Enlightenment when we thought that reason could explain the world. Then philosophers after the atrocities of the Second World War pointed out that such belief is really another kind of mythology itself. The mythology is the belief that we can achieve objective truth if we apply a certain methodology.

We could also say, "I don't really know, unless God tells me. I have to ask God and see what God says about it" – there are quite a few people who do exactly that. We can thus imagine replacing our reference to needing scientific evidence with a reference to *God* and it might be just as clever or silly as before.

ED: It's like the famous story, "I'm feeling much better thanks to God and to Dr. Brown and not necessarily in that order."

NADER: Rousseau would say something like, "Nature heals and the doctor sends the bill."

ED: I've been wrestling with all sorts of different things. I've been keeping a daily diary, which bounces around like a rubber ball. I assume that is good, because that's what we humans do – our minds wander over a wide range of possibilities.

NADER: I was just looking at pictures of a so-called healthy neuron and one that is not considered healthy. It's like a Rorschach test, "What do you want to see?"

When I see a so-called healthy neuron, I'm reminded of a young person with taut skin, no wrinkles, and rosy-colored cheeks. When you see this drawn, wrinkled neuron, I see something else. Wouldn't it be beautiful to find out what you would read into each picture? Let's say it wouldn't be about health and illness.

What do you see when you look at this picture of three old guys sitting together?

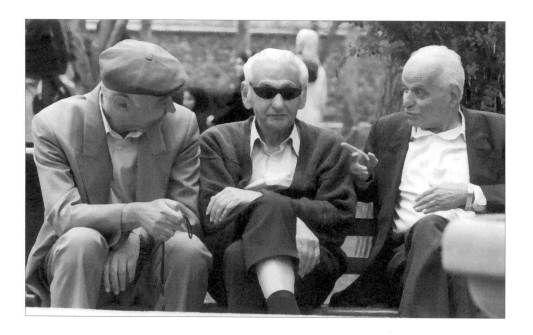

ED: They're beautiful. They are absolutely beautiful.

NADER: They appear calm. They do not seem hurried, in a rush, or tense.

ED: Maybe how we should describe elderhood is when we pass beyond the frantic race for life that occurs within the first 50 years. Then you finally catch on that life is not about being in a hurry. Life is about trying to care for yourself and those around you.

NADER: That feels right. So if you were looking at brain scans, what would you see? Suppose you saw holes, and big black spots. I look at this brain, look at the freedom therein, look at the space that has been made, look at the openness that has been created. What if we saw those black spots as gifts from the gods instead of thinking of protein deposits that have destroyed brain cells?

So these scans can be interpreted in a scientific way or from an artistic, a poetic point of view.

ED: Because it's the easiest conclusion doesn't mean it's the right conclusion.

NADER: It's not even the easiest; it's the mainstream because many of us are looking for so-called optimal functioning and often do not ask: why are we looking for it? What is so good about optimal functioning? Who or what is it for? I wonder what Gandhi's brain looked like? Or Mother Theresa's?

There was a study done on nuns. One nun showed symptoms of Alzheimer's, but her brain was classified as healthy. Another nun's brain looked like it was completely diseased according to some scientific understanding, but she didn't show any symptoms of Alzheimer's.

ED: Right now the trend is to do these brain games so that you can keep your brain healthy. They are saying our brains are not healthy, unless we do these games.

NADER: In some ways that is akin to our race for the optimal body. Often we live anxious, scared, and unrelated lives. We are lonely and isolated, but we have this perfectly operating body that we take to the gym for an hour a day, a brilliant humming machine, but the content of it is suffering.

ED: That's what my son is doing. Did I tell you about my son? My son is the president and general manager of a company that does glass replacement for car rental agencies. They operate in 20 states, so this week he was in Atlanta; the week before he was in New Jersey. He's not gone all the time, but he is frequently gone. He's also taking a graduate course in theology.

He and my daughter-in-law are marathon runners and they were just in New York to run in the New York City marathon. He is very busy and very driven.

My son is also a soccer coach for my granddaughter, who is a tough forward at the age of 10. And he will be running in the Los Angeles marathon with my granddaughter, who is 13. This will be her third marathon.

She hates it, but my son and daughter-in-law pressure her to do it, because it puts her in the class with a bunch of kids who are high producers, as if high production is the one goal in life.

NADER: The running away. Well, this gets back to achievement and performance measured by how many words I remember and how productive I am. So the person with Alzheimer's who seems to be just sitting around with some expression on his or her face is considered not fully human, somehow defective.

There is another point of view that all of us are part of a larger field. For example, in a group of people there are those who speak and those who don't. Those who don't speak are equally as important as those who do speak, because they are setting the mood, they are listening, they are holding. They're present and their energy influences the atmosphere as much as those who are assertive and clear in their articulations.

This reminds me of the question if you prefer an active, running-around lifestyle to the lifestyle of the old man who seems to just sit there. When we talk about the developed countries versus the non-developed countries, what do we mean? Developed in what way? When we talk about the Far East or Middle East — far or in the middle from what point? Who or what decides how we see the world?

"Maybe how we should describe elderhood is when we pass beyond the frantic race for life that occurs within the first 50 years."

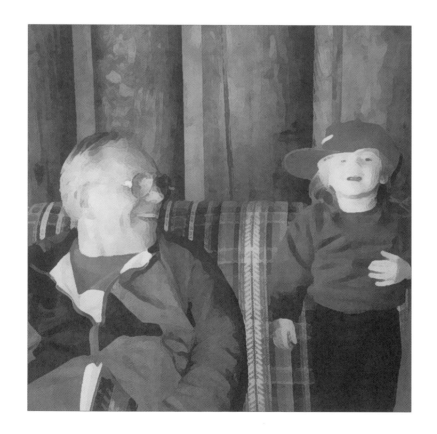

Chapter 9

When you're finished changing, you're finished.

— *Benjamin Franklin*

As We Live, We Change

Pat: Ed, have you developed techniques or ways of remembering things to adapt to the changes you have experienced? Like sometimes people will become careful about writing things down.

Ed: Because I'm keeping a diary, I write every day.

Pat: I was thinking more in terms of the mundane things. For example, I put everything back in my wallet the same way and I put my keys in the same spot when I get home, so I know where they're at.

I was talking with someone from Switzerland who did a qualitative study of people with forgetfulness in Switzerland. Some of the things people did were to make lists where they hadn't made lists before, or they put a basket by the front door of the house, and they always put their purse or their wallet or their keys in the basket. They used these techniques to create a way to jog their memory or to allow them to do things that in the past they wouldn't necessarily have had to think about. Do you do that at all?

ED: Yes. For example, I quit driving, and since I've quit driving I don't lose my car in the parking lot anymore.

PAT: That's a real good thing.

ED: Actually, there are a lot of things that I'm doing, because I do find that I'm losing things, and it's really frustrating. I was talking to a friend of mine a couple of days ago, and he was saying that more and more he loses more and more things. He was really frustrated, because he couldn't find his car keys. He's a really bright guy, but he said he was doing this more and more all the time.

I always put my keys here or I always put my keys there, but sometimes I don't know where I put them. So I have vowed that I am going to quit multitasking, because I'm doing my best with just one task at a time. But I have many friends who have the same problem who have not been diagnosed with dementia or Alzheimer's.

PAT: There is this idea of normal aging where we know we will begin to forget things. What you're talking about with your friends is that they are bemoaning the fact they can't remember as well as they once could.

I'm wondering whether we need to have a different perspective about that, because they are bemoaning and wishing for something that is not going to be there. In fact they, all of us, will probably become less able to remember things. We need to embrace that when we think about structuring our lives in ways that take that into account as we age.

Ed: Adaptation is what you're talking about?

Pat: Yes, acceptance of someone who is forgetful and changing the way the world is around us. But, unfortunately, we live in a larger structure that doesn't want to allow those changes to occur.

As people become forgetful, people who are the normal folks may not understand the world of the forgetful person. I wonder if that is a metaphor for the fear of things, like the fear of death, which, as far as we know in our corporeal world, is the ultimate transition to some other potential state of consciousness or total nothingness. And that's a scary thing.

Ed: I may be the king of denial, but the prospect of death has no fear for me, because it has no reality.

Nader: People don't tend to distinguish between death and dying.

Ed: Dying has little aspects to it; it's not one big aspect.

Nader: That's right. And I like what Pat said. If I'm so attached to my identity that is my name, my work, my job and where I live and what I have, and if there are cracks in that, I can really get into a panic. If I am not a professor anymore, what am I then? What if I had more fluidity? Let's say I'm also a lover and a playful kid irrespective of how old I am, and I'm a dreamer. Then, if there are some changes, it's not that much of a panic, because those changes create more room for something else. I can be more of a dreamer, because I'm less of a teacher. Or I can have different names, because I'm not so attached to one name.

PAT: I wonder if we as humans want to define ourselves in a particular way, not as fluid as we could be, but more static in the context of the social roles we occupy. "I am a community volunteer," or "I am a business executive," which we give different levels of status and prestige to, might be feeding our egos. As opposed to saying, "I am all these things and yet I'm none of these things."

Ed, you just expressed that death has no reality for you. What do you mean by that?

ED: I mean there's nothing practical to scare me about death now.

Years ago, a friend of mine had AIDS and this was before there were drugs to handle it. He was near death, so he talked to a mutual friend of ours and she took him down to the funeral parlor and he selected his casket. He selected the hors d'oeuvres to serve at his memorial and he helped prepare the memorial, so death had a reality to him.

The funeral parlor had a casket that was gray Naugahyde. He said, "I look great in gray, but not in Naugahyde." That is what I mean when I say I try and scare myself with what? What is there? I know it's going to happen. I just hope death is real quiet and sneaks up behind me and does it.

NADER: That's interesting, because you're on your own path, if you want to go there, but with death there is no identity to know. In some ways we have the spectrum between a static identity that I am my name and this body, to a complete nonidentity.

Certain spiritual traditions try to differentiate between different dimensions of reality and identity. There's the emotional identity and the spiritual identity. You are not only your body; it is just a part of who you are. You are your body, you are your memory, you are your experiences and you are probably more, much of which we don't yet understand.

PAT: It's interesting and also problematic. If we admit that we are biological creatures grounded in a physical reality, then we have to do things to exist as a biological creature and, at least in the world we know, that existence is intimately tied to the creation of these other ways of thinking like you just articulated.

It's a strange duality, because it's thinking about us as not purely physical or biological creatures but as something else beyond that. The concept of soul is one that humans have created to rise above the biological in this physical world.

The concepts of Alzheimer's disease are grounded in the biological substrate of the brain from the standpoint of trying to find a cure or treatment. That is the focus. But the human mind conceives of itself as a brain and then tries to act upon that based upon a biochemical understanding of connections, which is not the whole of what it means and what it is. And the distinction between those two is odd, because one is totally reductionistic to the biological, but does not phenomenologically capture the lived experience of forgetfulness.

It's odd the way we as a society have reduced it to those biological components. One could argue those biological concepts don't further the concept of how to accommodate people with forgetfulness in society. It is like, "Well, we'll give you some drugs." That becomes the way to deal with it – we give people medications. I wanted to ask you about that, Ed. A while back, you were saying how you felt the medication had helped you sustain your functioning. Do you still feel that way?

ED: Unquestionably. I really was in the fog last summer and I got the medication about the first of August, so I'm now approaching six months. I suspected I would have some slippage in the past two or three months, but a friend called me the other day and said, "I'm going to tell everybody you're a liar. You can't have Alzheimer's because you are too articulate."

Three times in the last week I felt that there was a tendency to say, "Everything that happens is Alzheimer's," which I know is not true. My cavities in my teeth have nothing to do with Alzheimer's, as far as I know. They have to do with my reluctance to go to the dentist. I ask myself, before Alzheimer's how would I have dealt with this; now post-Alzheimer's would it be the same way?

PAT: Your comment that you phenomenologically can perceive a difference with the medication is interesting. That would be a testimonial in favor of the concept that there is a biological thing going on that is changeable to some extent from the standpoint of body chemistry, which is fine. But it seems like we have to get more balanced to where it's not just drugs, it is other ways that are more interactional and social, in terms of preparing ourselves for these types of events that we will all experience from the standpoint of forgetfulness.

Nader, since you are a therapist familiar with the terminology, is hallucination seeing or hearing something that isn't there? And if something is there but you misidentify it, what is that? Is that a delusion?

NADER: Yes, that's a good definition. But from the paradigm I come from, there are no hallucinations. You spoke earlier about how there is a basic substrate called reality. From that point of view, you could say that if there were something that did not concur with that reality, we would need to call it a hallucination. But as we know from quantum physics, shamanism and other approaches of looking at life, they are just different, parallel worlds.

PAT: It's interesting that the psychiatric category of hallucinations and delusions is a way of labeling alternative views of reality that don't fit into the dominant mode of the way things should be. That then provides a justification for certain types of treatments or sanctions against the individual. And that mechanism is socially controlled. Something is done with medications, for example.

NADER: Social control means we want to make sure that you stay within the way we have defined reality. We outlaw any mind-altering substances. We criminalize what poses a threat to our agreed-upon reality. I am wondering why these other realities are so scary to many of us? Why are we not simply curious about those other realities and ways of being?

PAT: So as we live we change, but others want to conceive of us as something that we are no longer. Sometimes people change in ways that we can't conceive of, and sometimes it's hard to accept those changes.

NADER: Imagine living within a social climate that has much more fluidity around what we expect of a person's behavior. For example, if I talk and I am able to get words out, that ability to be verbal is often related in our society to intelligence, presentability, assertiveness, smarts, and all of that.

Imagine living in a society where all these different expressions are amazing expressions and I don't have to judge you. You speak differently than he does, but there is no judgment around other than, "You could be an artist," "You could be a farmer," or "You could have Alzheimer's." There is an absence of hierarchy and valuation.

Remember that the ancient Greeks use the word *zenos* to refer to both stranger and friend, foreigner and ally – a nice example of an attitude that is welcoming to what is new, strange and/or different.

"I quit driving, and since I've quit driving, I don't lose my car in the parking lot anymore."

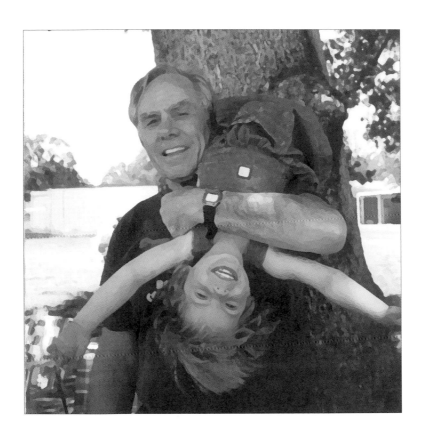

Chapter 10

The longer I live, the more beautiful life becomes.

— *Frank Lloyd Wright*

The Essence of Ageism

Ed: One of the things I was uninformed about until this occurred was anti-elder bias. "Anti" is probably too strong a word, but elders are not considered people, and now I'm one of them!

People like me who have become acclimated to elderhood discover that there is a terribly subtle bias. It's like I don't have anything to contribute that anyone wants.

I mentioned to you earlier the terrors of my love life. I've been going through this thing with my girlfriend and we came to the parting of our ways since I last saw you.

I have a good friend. We've been friends for 20 years. We were talking about my girlfriend and me splitting. I was speculating on some reasons and he said, "You're too old," like I was a tooth that needed to be replaced.

What the hell does "too old" mean? Too old for what? But I didn't challenge him. He's a good friend and he was not attacking me. He was just saying I'm not the guy I once was. And I see it in lots of other settings. Most of them are so subtle it's almost impossible to attribute it directly to any one thing, but it is there.

I have thought about writing a book about it and entitling it *Not Dead Yet*. I've been working constantly, since I was 16, but now I've reached the point where society says, "He's waste product. Let's move him out of the way and not let him block progress." And I'm really upset about it.

PAT: That has been called ageism. Sexism, racism, and ageism are pervasive in our society. You touched on part of it when you were talking about how you were part of the paid work force since you were 16. And for men especially, what you do for work is a central component of identity. It is also a central component of other people's conception of somebody who is productive and who Ed is. But upon retirement there's a transition and you're out of that system.

It goes even beyond that. Like I said earlier, in prior times the idea of death was this mysterious thing. It was a force from outside that came and took people away and there wasn't a clear explanation for it. But in our modern times that has been reduced to biological functioning of the body to where death occurs, not because of some mysterious force, but because of cellular processes or wear and tear.

That takes the mystery out of it and tries to put it down to something primarily in the biological world. And it's not that this is unimportant, but it tends to dominate our thinking about our growing older. It's called the bio-medicalization of aging, where we look at the body as the source of aging and we neglect the meaning of aging in a larger context.

I think that's what happens when people see a person as an older person. There are these stereotypes that discount that person without even encountering that person. That is the essence of ageism.

I wanted to go back to where you were talking about your relationship breakdown with your girlfriend. What is the difference in age between you and her?

ED: I'm 73. She's 61. She and I had been together for four years. And if I had to pin it down, I would say the relationship broke up because of my careless behavior rather than her dropping me, because I got angry at her and quit seeing her for some time.

Then she pursued me rather than my pursuing her. I was cavalier about it. I spent two years in Orange County and it was during that time that she met another guy. If she was so damn important, I should have been there and paid some attention and it probably wouldn't have happened.

PAT: Do you think she was worried about your Alzheimer's and what that might lead to?

ED: It's hard to say, but her mother had Alzheimer's so she is familiar with it. When I became aware of the fact that I had it and shared that with her, if anything it heightened her interest in me at least on a day-to-day basis. But it may have also done the same thing that ageism does. It may have pushed me over into another category.

She and I had a compatible relationship. Even when I was in Orange County, I seldom went more than a couple days where I didn't get an e-mail from her. So we had a very strong connection. Yet, I can see how women who were attracted to me a year or two ago might not be attracted to me so much today. But I haven't had an opportunity to test that theory.

NADER: I remember this Hollywood movie. There was something very moving about its simple plot line where a couple in love experiences tragedy. The man gets run over by a car, dies, but not quite; his spirit is still a little bit on earth. He can't quite leave this life, because there's something he's still missing.

As the movie unfolds, you learn how he wants to give his girlfriend one last kiss, to feel that human touch. I think about that as an appreciation for the fact that we are alive, because often in spiritual traditions – perhaps misunderstood by us – there is an emphasis on, "Let's get this life over with so we can be up in nirvana land."

I am not sure I really appreciate the wonder of human touch, to feel and to make contact that way. What it feels like to touch somebody else's skin for a moment. Then, the metaphor of a kiss, the intimate sharing that entails so much before that kiss can happen. There has to be intimate divineness to make that contact.

ED: When I kissed my girlfriend goodbye, there was that special moment. It is a privilege to be present to these things.

It also occurred to me that it is very easy to say I got caught by the red light that was an Alzheimer's reminder, that whatever I'm experiencing in my life is suddenly going to be delegated to Alzheimer's.

NADER: The lens through which you see things?

ED: You could make a note of that if you want. Anything I did wrong was caused by Alzheimer's. Don't forget it either.

"What the hell does "too old" mean? Too old for what?"

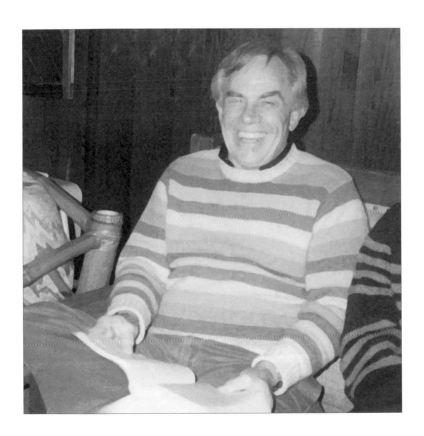

Chapter **11**

I HAVE GREAT FAITH IN FOOLS; SELF-CONFIDENCE MY FRIENDS CALL IT.

— *EDGAR ALLAN POE*

WHAT'S SO GOOD ABOUT CONFIDENCE?

ED: When my doctor sent me this letter saying, "Ed, you've got dementia," I thought, "You mean you think I lost my mind?"

NADER: Finally.

ED: Thought I'd never get rid of that damn thing.

NADER: God, it's been giving me a headache so much of the time!

ED: Then I got this medication to take and things started to change.

NADER: Do you still feel the forgetfulness of the dementia somewhere?

ED: Unquestionably, I feel it. These are sensations I've never had. I don't know how to explain it, except that I'm aware of a lack of self-confidence that I've never had before. I feel a weakness in not being able to do things I was able to do before and I don't know how to assess my limits.

Nader: Help me understand what you mean by confidence. What is that?

Ed: Well, mostly I've been a builder. And the ultimate challenge when I was undertaking a project was that I had to be able to say to you, "Nader, there are a lot of questions here, and we'll solve them together, but I will finish the project. We will stick with this until we get it done."

The only way I know to explain it is that there was that innate sense that I've done this. I have been involved in the building of probably 4,000 units of housing. So when I came to unit 4,001, I could look back and say, "I've been doing it for this long. I've faced a lot of problems, but I've been able to work my way through."

So I'm able to say to you, "Nader, we can do this project. We have the financial capacity and the crew capacity," and so forth. And now I really do not know how to say I can do anything. That's because I realize there is a trapdoor that is going to drop and I'm going to go shooting through it.

Nader: And you don't know which one or where it is.

Ed: And I don't know how long it'll be, but I do know it will come.

Nader: You are speaking from this place called normality, "The Ed that I know." What if I were to say, "There is also the Ed that I don't know?"

And from that position, what would that Ed say about what you call lack of confidence?

Or, put another way, if there is Ed who looks at the "normal" Ed from one point of view, then there's also a different Ed that you're becoming in some ways. We could say that we're always becoming, but it's more pronounced right now for you because it's not so subtle. And on this road to the Ed who you are becoming, the one who has less confidence, what would he say to the normal Ed?

ED: What if I were to say that life has infinite possibilities and life's challenge is to invite me to explore where I can go? Maybe I can't do it, but one thing I have learned in life is that we don't do anything by ourselves, so it's important for me to be open to be in relationship with other people and to try to open doors.

When I discovered I had Alzheimer's or dementia or both, I tried to get help from the Alzheimer's Association and others and the uniform response was, "Where is your family member or caregiver?" I had no authority of my own any longer.

I've been self-sufficient all my life. I've been a businessman and I've been in management all my life. So I'm not inclined to sit back and say, "I've got Alzheimer's. I can't do anything." I have Alzheimer's but I know I can do something. I know I can contribute somewhere.

NADER: At breakfast this morning, you were talking about your joyous moment appreciating the sun, the golden globe and the diversity of people, including the person who was homeless covered with six blankets, because he was cold. Using that example, we could say we all live in different realities, but that doesn't preclude us from experiencing the joy of life.

ED: With one another.

NADER: With one another, connected to the homeless person or you on your own at that moment and relaying all of it. No matter how different the realities are, it's up to us how we perceive what is around us.

From the point of view of the new reality you are entering, you feel a lack of confidence. We can, of course, look through the paradigm of loss, but we can also say, "What's so good about confidence?" In our normal world it's highly touted.

ED: It's essential.

NADER: Yet, in some imaginary other world, for example, confidence might mean arrogance. It would mean that you have forgotten that we live in an interconnected universe.

ED: And that means no possibility of separate confidence, because it can only come through groups.

NADER: Exactly. Then you can say that it is arrogant to say, "I have confidence." Confidence? An earthquake could happen this very second and here you are who has just proclaimed, "I have the confidence to build a skyscraper." Your project is leveled to rubble by forces way out of your control. So confidence from that point of view could be seen as a character flaw. Your idea of "I have confidence" might just be an illusory way of looking at life.

ED: Well, confidence usually means I can do it myself. So I don't need you.

NADER: That sounds like one of the definitions of the rugged individualist we seem to value so highly in this culture.

ED: It means I've got this thing under control. Just stick around, and I'll show you control.

NADER: I'm the big cheese.

ED: I could tell you a couple stories that would curl your hair.

NADER: Expressions of confidence, you mean?

ED: Of moments when I had absolute confidence I could do anything. But that just shows how many things I had never thought of.

NADER: The gods sheltered you from all the possibilities.

ED: And then they turned it loose like a Brazilian rainstorm. It was a painful lesson in reality: "Welcome back to the world, Ed, welcome back."

I was a safety officer of my squadron and it was my challenge to help the other pilots to be aware of reality, because if there is a cockier group on earth than Navy pilots, I don't know who they are. And I was introduced to this story that demonstrated their reality.

They said almost anybody could handle a mechanical failure in their plane, because there are all kinds of safety measures to deal with that. If you have two systems fall apart at the same time, that's much more difficult. And if you get three at one time, it's almost impossible. If you get four, kiss your ass goodbye!

In the things that I recall, I did have the absolute confidence I could handle everything. And then on this one project, my superintendent lied and signed off things as completed he had never done. It was deliberate sabotage of the job. You know what? No one felt sorry for me. I said I could do it. I had the confidence I could do it, but then it just went on and on, one thing after another after another. Welcome to life, Ed.

NADER: It's almost like life is out there to give you a lesson. Not in a vindictive way, but for changing, for becoming more aware.

ED: I talked about the pilot who has one system blow out, no problem; two systems, probably okay; three, he can maybe make it; and four, he's gone. The reverse of that is the average successful businessperson who thinks that he or she did it all him or herself. How come everything went right for you and people came and supported you and gave you special consideration? Was that your skill or was that life giving you an opportunity to work successfully with other people?

When I received the information from my doctor that I had dementia, I was about as low as a snake's neck. But then it's been one generous thing after another. Bob came to me and said, "I don't know what I can do, but I would be happy to do anything that I could to help." And another friend said, "You're welcome to stay here," and he takes me to the bus stop. I could list endlessly all of the ways that people have reached out to me.

Before, I was self-sufficient. I didn't need them. I was confident I could do everything by myself. I can't imagine life being any richer than it is for me right now, because I have so many friends.

"When I received the information from my doctor that I had dementia, I was about as low as a snake's neck. But then it's been one generous thing after another."

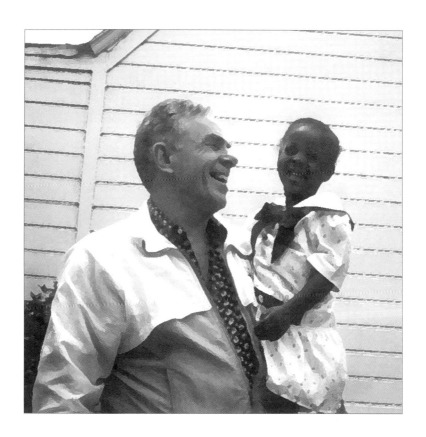

Chapter 12

Then there is the man who drowned crossing a stream with an average depth of six inches.

— *W.I.F. Gates*

Statistical (Wo)man Does Not Exist

Ed: I read something that said people who use their minds for various detailed things often don't show symptoms of Alzheimer's. There was a story of one very bright guy who died. They decided to do an autopsy to look at his brain and see if there was anything special. And he had Alzheimer's, but he had not shown the symptoms.

Pat: In the history of Alzheimer's disease that was one of the complicating factors. They would do autopsies on people who they thought had Alzheimer's and they'd find no sign of it. Then they'd do autopsies on elderly people who died and didn't show any dementia and they would find pathological evidence of Alzheimer's disease.

Nader: It gets back to the nun study where they saw the same phenomenon. Even though this nun's brain was 90 percent unused, there were no manifestations that she had Alzheimer's.

I'm wondering if it was because the nun was in the atmosphere of a nunnery where different priorities are set. In a nunnery you are much more regarded if you can have the ability to be silent, the ability to relate nonverbally. Speaking is not awarded a high status. One's ability to keep or stay quiet is seen as an important skill.

PAT: When the nuns came into the order they had to write an essay and researchers looked at them. They looked at the content and the complexity of how language was used and they found a correlation between how people used their brains and how well they did on the essays.

I think this was what you were talking about earlier, Ed, this idea of a reserve where if you do a lot of things in your life – if you're a scientist or you do something where you use your brain a lot – the neurological pathways become more complex and intertwined. So when there are insults physiologically to the brain pathology there are other pathways, other roads that you can compensate for.

At an academic medical center I visited they talked about two sisters who came in for evaluation for memory. And if you looked at the neurocognitive testing, the sister who didn't appear to be demented had much worse scores than the sister who appeared to be much more demented.

ED: Why was that?

PAT: The sister who did not appear to be demented manifested very few observable symptoms because of her ability to compensate for what she couldn't remember by using humor, by being gregarious, by engaging people.

They said – and these are people for whom this is their stock-in-trade – it was amazing when you looked at the empirical data derived from the clinical examinations, because you would think this woman would be the much more acute case, but in fact it was the opposite.

It's odd how we create these constructs that people supposedly can fit under and maybe most people do, but it doesn't tell you what's going to happen to any individual person's case. It's the old idea that the statistical man or woman does not exist.

It's also interesting that Alzheimer's was once conceived of as not affecting older people but as affecting younger people. And when you got old, you had senile dementia.

NADER: I have become so sensitive about diagnosing symptoms and have developed an adverse feeling towards it because of diagnostic fads and trends. It seems that in the last 50 years every decade since had some hip diagnostic label, whether it was neurosis, schizophrenia, borderline, anxiety disorder, or whatever.

PAT: What's interesting about psychiatry and psychology from a sociological perspective is that it's a mechanism for social control, for defining classes of people.

What's interesting about European history is that, especially in England, the church would care for people with mental infirmities. Then there was the rise of psychiatry where they claimed that, based on science, they would be able to find the problems in someone's head.

That's where Alzheimer was coming from – "Let's look at the pathology and let's correlate that with the behavior" – and somehow there was a leap of faith, and it's still strong. Freud came out of that, but he couldn't find really a connection between the two. And then the psychodynamic model arose. Now, it's getting back to the biological basis, but it's not new. The techniques are new, but it's the same way of trying to answer the questions as to why people are different.

NADER: Freud was a neuroscientist. He wanted to reduce psychological symptoms to neurophysiology, very much akin to today's bio-psychiatrists. Yet, Freud, deep down, was also a humanist, could see that it was too simplistic to believe that everything was reducible to neurons. Actually, his theory was quite different from his therapeutic practice. From those who knew him and from some of his writings you get the feeling that he was so very human, present and heartfelt with his clients.

So it is a challenge to keep an open mind, to keep in abeyance the idea that anything that's happening is happening because of some given diagnosis. How do we enlarge the medical paradigm?

ED: There are a lot of other new phenomena in my life that clearly have nothing to do with Alzheimer's. So it seems to me that I should simply report the things that happen to me without trying to tell you how they happened. If you find me lying in the street, it doesn't mean I was run over by a car.

NADER: That's right.

ED: Just catching a nap here.

NADER: A new way to meet someone.

PAT: Unless you want tire marks on your shirt.

NADER: The power of the image of what is a normal life: that I behave in a certain way, that I do certain things. And if I don't, what is going on?

We have so much opportunity with forgetfulness and with what is called mental illness. These differences from our "normality" present us with other realities and ways of being that can truly deepen us. They make us aware of our expectations, how we are trapped in our customary ways of being. I expect Ed to do this and that, and if that's not happening, then what do I do? Either I say, "Ed is nuts and I'm going to avoid him," or I am curious and deepen my understanding of his reality and therefore of my own.

PAT: There is this concept coming out of supporting "neurological diversity."

Remember the video you sent me, Nader? The one where this woman who is autistic has a machine where she can type in her thoughts? She was sitting there doing all these things that from the normative standpoint one would think, "Wow, she is really out in limbo."

Writing about what she was doing, she said, "I'm interacting with my world in a way where I'm really getting into what's happening around me, and you folks don't do this. I look at patterns and I see things."

NADER: That's right. She held her hands under running water and it looked like she was lost in that water, but then her explanation through the computer interface was, "I'm feeling the water. I'm interacting with the water and I'm taking my time with that."

So where at first it looked like she is so very strange, suddenly what she was doing had meaning, and the person who is really strange is me. I instrumentalized water for my purposes and forgot how much more there is to water than how I use it.

PAT: If society allowed that kind of diversity to flourish, you could magically change something that is generally seen as meaningless into something that has meaning. I would bet that people won't do that, though, because the world is organized around competition that becomes the way of life. If you don't adopt it, you start to see your whole world slide away. And that is so powerful, because then everybody does it, and if you don't do it, you're not going to be around.

NADER: You think of how our economic system burdens us and then you see somebody in Africa barely scraping by. So in some ways that eight-to-five job would look good from the point of view of an African life. It goes back to remembering how our attitude can determine how we see the world and how we experience it.

That reminds me of a beautiful story. We had a new resident coming to our care home. A beautiful 92-year-old woman in a wheelchair was brought into the lobby of our assisted-living community. I happened to be present at that time so I said to her, "Ms. Jones, thanks for coming. How are you?" She was a very chipper, tiny woman, and she said, "Oh, I'm fine."

I said, "Ms. Jones, I would love to show you your room to make sure you like it." And Ms. Jones looked at me and said, "Oh, no worries. I've already made up my mind that I will like it."

"I've been self-sufficient all my life. I've been a business-man and I've been in management all my life. So I'm not inclined to sit back and say, 'I've got Alzheimer's. I can't do anything.'"

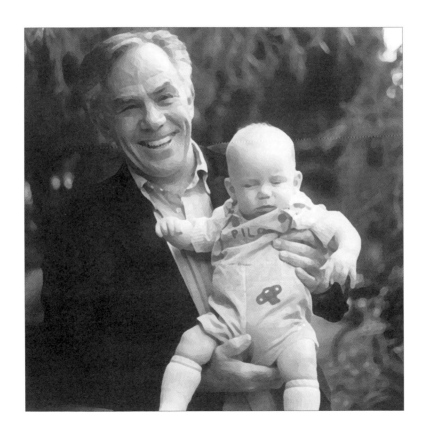

Chapter **13**

Do I contradict myself? Very well then, I contradict myself.

— *Walt Whitman*

Waiting for Forgetfulness

Nader: A fundamental philosophical question is: Why is there something rather than nothing? What does it mean to live a human life?

There are other questions: Whose life am I living – a life that follows the images given by the society in which I live? Or is life coming out of me and I am authenticated in that? Of course, authenticity is a construct itself. Does anyone really know what it means to be "authentic"? Who or what determines what is "authentic" anyway?

Somehow whatever symptom I experience is not desirable because it disorganizes me. On the other hand, symptoms are desirable because they shake me up and allow me to have a glimpse of another world – anything to break out of ordinary states of consciousness.

Then the question becomes: If human life is that one moment of awakening, would that make life worth living? That's one viewpoint.

James Hillman points out that symptoms want to be tended to; they want tender loving care. You could say that the symptom I am experiencing is pushing me to be more loving, more aware of who I am.

Toward the end of Oedipus' life, after some 90 years, he basically says, "All that suffering I have undergone – killing my dad, marrying my mother, having two kids, being the king, suffering the destruction of my city and my kingdom, and now being blind and being led around by my daughter – all of that was worth it. Why? Because I learned to love." That is one viewpoint.

Waiting for forgetfulness – that is a provocative statement. Yet, from the place I am coming from, I see little difference to other statements I would make, all of which sound more acceptable to many of us. For example, you might say: waiting to wake up; waiting to see other ways of living; waiting to experience something that gets me to live with more awareness.

We have been talking about the fact that if I'm lucky enough to be within an environment that appreciates my suffering and symptom, then I may have it made. But if I'm not, then it could be agony.

PAT: Some people talk about dementia and the moral responsibility of society to ensure that people who are forgetful can live in the world in a reasonably human and just way. So, how can we create a cultural space wherein that phenomenon, however it's expressed, can be supported and not be denigrated or dehumanized in terms of the way people who are forgetful are treated by the rest of the world? Or in practical terms, can we create a world that is more "forgetfulness friendly?"

If you think about it in those terms, it's an idea that there are all kinds of ways of being that we accommodate for one reason or another. A good example is children who are born with Down syndrome. We create protective work environments and centers to attend to their needs. It's a way of thinking that is more conscious about the things that we deal with and must deal with as a society. But there are no pathways for dementia, because we don't think about it in the way you just described it. We think about it primarily in terms of a negative loss kind of mentality.

It goes back to the question: If we have an attitudinal change toward dementia, where does that lead us? We talk about it. We think it's a good thing to pursue, but it's not clear how we do that.

NADER: We just had our curbs torn up in our neighborhood, because they were putting in ramps. They are for wheelchairs. Today you find also more and more stoplights where you hear a bird chirping away so people who are blind can navigate the streets on their own. Braille is more and more present so we are adapting to other ways of being. These are first steps to come to terms with difference from some norm.

PAT: If we can accommodate these other things that are being accommodated, like curb cuts for wheelchairs or chirping noises for visually impaired people, then maybe we can prepare for the aging or the graying of our society. If we think of forgetfulness as an archetype, if we can make room for that, then maybe other things will follow.

NADER: Yes, along with an ever-deepening acceptance, perhaps even welcoming.

ED: I worry about myself sometimes in that I conclude that — because it seems real to me yet not present at the current time — the image is the reality. It will become who we are as a planet at some time in the future — dinosaurs rolling over so I can scratch their tummies. My hopeful brain may not be entirely trustworthy, but nevertheless I feel the presence of this thought in my mind, meaning it is real and that it's not my responsibility to worry about it, only to accommodate it as much and as deeply as I am capable in my life at this time.

I believe the spirit of life will take it to where it needs to, and maybe it won't be while I'm here, but that's why I find it exciting. It's like in a marathon, as you're racing toward the finish line. I have no idea how far we are from the finish line. I'm not sure, if it's 26.3 miles or .3 miles, but nevertheless I get to be in the race. I get to experience the excitement of seeing change.

NADER: I like the idea of people accepting that forgetfulness is part of our life and that at one point much of what we have learned in a consensus world will be forgotten. Then we will be pushed to feel through to what else is important, that it is not only about knowing the elementary table or how to build a house. That brings us back to the fundamental question of: What makes us human?

I had this friend, Elizabeth. Her husband was a very accomplished author and psychologist. At 92 years of age, he didn't remember the books he's written, and that he was one of the well-known American psychologists of the last 50 years or so.

While he had forgotten his books, the two things he did remember and constantly repeated to his wife were "I love you," and "You are so beautiful." What more can you want? He forgot most things but remembered to say what mattered to him most.

When people asked her, "How is it to be with Jim?" she said, "I love it. It couldn't get any better than this." Because if we are going to forget all the stuff that we're amassing right now, what matters then, really?

Pat: Let's say for the sake of discussion that you forgot and did not have a sense of past or future. Would you then be in the present but you are not worrying about it because everybody around you is worrying about it?

That's what I was asking earlier: "Can we create a cultural space for this?" What if you had this Bio-Dome and people could say, "This is where you go, if you don't remember anything, because the world is structured to where you don't have to remember anything. It doesn't matter whether you remember, you don't have to." What would that world look like?

Nader: As we are moving deeper into the information age, there is a counter movement that says, "Hey, wait a minute. Yes, it is about more giga and tetra-bytes, but it's also about awareness. As I'm running through life, I see that infamous flower, and it reminds me for a second that there is something else."

I have a friend who calls me. The first thing he says is, "Breathe." And I suddenly remember life is bigger than my 50 items on the task list. I sit down and make a cup of tea and all of that has space rather than what we usually do, which is to say, "This doesn't belong here." We put you in an adult-only community when you get older. We put you in a dementia clinic when you get dementia. And when you're dying, we put you in Ward Number Five.

We keep our life nice and pristine, so there's no impediment as we're running from one place to another. There is no reminder of other realities. And these homeless people really grate on us, because they take away from our manicured environment.

ED: When you start talking with homeless people you are often surprised about their vitality.

NADER: Most people don't see it that way. They see homeless people and say, "We need to take care of that problem because they are bothering us. They are disturbing the flow. They are panhandling. They're even getting aggressive."

PAT: You'd think they were starving or something! That's what we do. We keep people away whether it's based on skin color, religion, or cognitive capacity. We're always keeping people separate.

I like the idea you came up with, Nader, about love being important, because it is the most powerful thing, but it is something we don't use much in our everyday lives for whatever reason.

ED: It's been my experience as a fund-raiser that people do want to be part of organizations that are doing good things, but they don't want to be screwed for two cents. They are willing to let hundreds of opportunities go by so they don't get screwed by some huckster.

PAT: That's the fear about not expressing the love.

ED: The question about love is, "If I want love, how much is it going to cost me, because there is a finite supply?" Artificial scarcity has been the problem for human society throughout our times. "If I share my bone with you tonight, how do I know you'll have a bone to share with me tomorrow night?"

PAT: But if you don't remember, then you don't remember that you may not have a bone.

ED: You don't worry.

NADER: That's right. Then you are finally open to love.

PAT: It is interesting being around people with Down syndrome, because they show affection and unrestrained emotion toward others. In the Alzheimer's world, people want a cure because of the transition from the norm to the not-norm. In the Down's world, parents don't want a cure. They're afraid of a cure, because they think it will take away the essence of their child. Their children are not the norm but they're real, and they bring a reality that is not there to anybody else, and it's a refreshing reality.

It's an interesting juxtaposition of a person who always was one way and "we want to preserve that even though what the person is, is not the norm," versus "what they were is what we pine for, because they've become something that was not what we thought they were or would become."

ED: I don't know whether it's true of everybody, but all my life I've had a jukebox playing in my head. In the 1960s, my brain played Bob Dylan. I was not conscious of it until recently, but then I noticed that the music is going backward counter-wise. This morning some Bing Crosby music from the 1940s was playing. I don't remember the last time I listened to Bing Crosby in my brain. I was shocked he was there.

I'm wondering if this is a sign of the progression in my brain that these songs are playing and that they are from very long ago? I don't even remember listening to this stuff. I just wake up and Bing Crosby is singing, "How are things in Glacamora?" And I think, Gosh, I don't even remember where Glacamora is.

PAT: In the clinical characterization of Alzheimer's disease, the idea is that your short-term memory starts to go first, but you retain long-term memory.

ED: If you want to make any requests, let me know.

PAT: In-A-Gadda-Da-Vida.

ED: It's two bits a song.

PAT: We've been talking for a while now. Maybe it's time to break for lunch.

ED: The lunches are good, but the breakfasts are better.

"The question about love is, 'If I want love, how much is it going to cost me, because there is a finite supply?'"

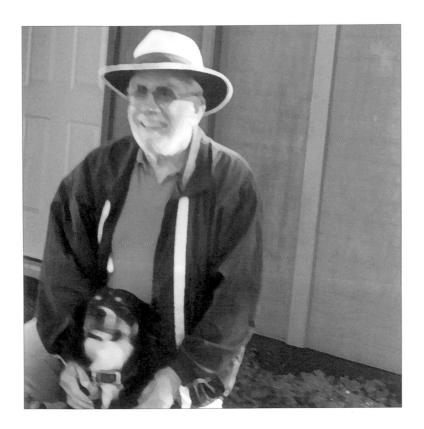

SOME FINAL THOUGHTS

Through the conversations with Ed, we hope to contribute to expanding the horizons of what forgetfulness can mean beyond loss, which we feel has yet to be actively sought in our society. Such an open horizon challenges our normative conceptions of forgetfulness, dementia, memory, personhood, aging and time.

Our understanding of personal and social growth is embedded within a dominant framework of striving for more – more outcomes, more memory, more years to live. From this notion of gain, it is fair to assert that loss is anything that prevents us from reaching outcomes – from accomplishing, from being engaged in work, from remaining youthful achievers. Forgetfulness falls on the loss side of this equation.

Alzheimer's disease is caused by various changes that result in so-called damaged brain cells. In the public it is predominantly defined by its symptoms and interpreted as the decline and final loss of memory and other cognitive abilities. Many of us might place most, if not all, of our hopes on finding a treatment and ultimately a cure for Alzheimer's disease.

But the fruits of such an approach are elusive and difficult to obtain, and no clear timetable can be set for harvesting the fruits of this belief. What if, in spite of all the best efforts of those conducting research into treatment and cures, these goals remain elusive into the foreseeable future? How do we care for people who are different from our expectations of what is normal, and what does that mean in terms of a philosophy of care? Do we treat them as diseased? Would that imply a certain derogatory stance toward the people for whom we care about? Or do we approach forgetful people with an attitude of respect, kindness, and acceptance of who they are in their new realities? Certainly, our dear friend Ed keeps appreciating the fact that we look at him as a full human being; lest we forget, he would surely let us know!

Just think for a moment: how does your attitude change if you know you are approaching someone you think is your teacher versus if you are approaching someone you think is diseased, cognitively impaired? We are very sensitive people and can sense the attitude behind those who care for us - whether we are forgetful or not. A central question thus becomes: How would you like to be approached if you were forgetful? What would you like the eyes to see that look at you?

Some argue that even if substantial therapeutic advances will be available in the near future, they may not be robust enough to slow the progression of forgetfulness among the many people who are experiencing cognitive changes as they age. The unfortunate by-product of the belief in the discovery of a cure is that we have not begun thinking about ways that our society can see forgetfulness as something more than a demon to be exorcised by a hoped-for medical treatment. Yet, rather than a debilitating disease that leaves those afflicted in a sad and lamentable state of existence, dementia may be another, altered state of consciousness, as valuable and important as our everyday or "normal" way of being. This requires, foremost, a curiosity, an openness to all that is, to look at forgetfulness, as it is, not in the way we believe to know it.

By engaging people to think about forgetfulness in the context of a wider horizon of possibilities, social change is possible. We may reduce the social stigma that people labeled with Alzheimer's disease experience. In that way we may not only accept and help others who are forgetful, but we may also be better prepared for our own inevitable forgetfulness. We believe it is time for society to think about and act toward forgetfulness and forgetful people in ways that may be currently unthinkable, but perhaps will become a reality in the future. Instead of being a crisis, forgetfulness may one day soon present an opportunity for knowing and deepening who we are.

Similarly, the issue of forgetfulness relates closely to the process of aging all of us experience. To live is to age, to age is to live. We cannot have it otherwise. To fear aging is to fear life itself. Yet, so many of us feel burdened by the many negative associations connected to aging and growing older. The decline metaphors we relate to aging, however, are based on some normative view of optimal health and functioning, a view that marginalizes important dimensions of life only possible through time and experience.

As with our needed attitudinal change towards forgetfulness, it is crucial that we change our perception of aging to one that understands its importance for deepening our maturation and eldership. Such eldership is of vital importance as we face the many challenges with which planet and people confront us today. It is from the perspective of the elder that we can ground our hope for transformation and change of our behavior toward our planet and fellow humans. Such behavior and attitude needs to be based on an understanding of how deeply planet and people are interconnected, how we inhabit a living universe on whose health our own is dependent. This knowledge forms part of the wisdom our elders hold and which our collective societies need to implement more urgently than ever.

ACKNOWLEDGEMENTS

We thank Bob Levitt, who was a friend of Ed and introduced Nader and Pat to him so we could begin this journey.

We would also like to thank Dr. Katja Reuter, Dr. Norman Fineman and Alan Klaum for their help in making the book more readable, to Paula Hertel and sister Elke Tekin for their constant encouragement and support, to Peggy Nauts for proof-reading, to Flora Cortez for her organizational help, to Geoffrey Faustman for his technical assistance in recording the conversations with Ed, to Bill Burton for his amazing knowledge of ancient Greek, to Tobie Smith and Finley Kipp for being so creative with the book's layout and pictures, and to Kluska, our AgeSong cocker spaniel, for her patience in waiting for her walks.

A big thank you to all of our friends and colleagues in academia, institutes, and organizations dedicated to helping our elders live respected and meaningful lives, especially to our residents at the AgeSong Senior Communities and many other elders we have met on our journeys – they have been our greatest teachers throughout the last few decades. Special thanks go also to our Pacific Institute interns as well as the staff at AgeSong and AgeSong at Bayside Park, who believed in our vision and our desire to change the view on aging, whose continued enthusiasm for the work with elders in various states of consciousness provide much of the inspiration and push behind this book.

Of course, without the support of our spouses, this book would not have been possible. Thanks to Ladan Ghashghaeipour, Nader's adorable wife, for her tireless encouragement and belief in the importance of this book, her deep knowing of the wisdom of the soul. And thanks to Sabrina Watson-Fox, Pat's loving wife — her wise insights about aging and life provided confirmation of the necessity for our discussions as a counter to ageist attitudes that are all too pervasive in our society.

The Authors

Ed Voris is a native of Dallas, Texas, where he graduated from Southern Methodist University with a Bachelor of Business Administration. He also received a Bachelor of Divinity from Conservative Baptist Theological Seminary in Denver, Colorado.

Following graduation he entered the construction industry with a principal interest in affordable housing; working in Texas, Washington and Hawaii. In 1986 Voris moved to Berkeley, California, for ongoing study at the Graduate Theological Union, where he joined the staff of the Center for Ethics and Social Policy. There Ed served as Organizing Editor of "A Cry for Justice," a study of the Economic Justice statements of the major religious bodies, published by Paulist Press.

Since then Ed has been a consultant to community development non-profits, specializing in housing and finance.

He was recently diagnosed with dementia.

Nader Robert Shabahangi, Ph.D. received his Doctorate degree from Stanford University, is a licensed psychotherapist and businessman. His multicultural background has made him an advocate for different marginalized groups of society throughout his adult life. In the 1980's he worked with abused children and teenagers and led anticipatory bereavement groups for Coming Home Hospice. In 1993 he founded the non-profit organization Pacific Institute with the purpose of training psychotherapists in a multicultural, humanistic approach to counseling and to provide affordable therapy services to the many diverse groups living in San Francisco. In 1994, noticing the often inhumane treatment of the elderly living in institutions, he started to develop an innovative Gerontological Wellness Program in order to provide emotional support and mental health care services for the elderly. In 1995, together with his two brothers, Nader started AgeSong, a company that develops and operates assisted living communities in the San Francisco Bay Area. Passionate about training therapists in a process-oriented, existential approach to working with people in need of care, he co-founded the Existential-Humanistic Institute in 1997. In 2002 he founded Elders Academy Press, a publishing program of Pacific Institute and Pacific Institute Europe, specifically dedicated to promoting writings of and for elders. In 2003 Nader wrote *Faces of Aging* as a tribute and celebration of growing old and being an elder. In 2008 he co-authored *Deeper into the Soul*, a book aimed at de-stigmatizing and at broadening our understanding of dementia.

[www.agesong.com and www.pacificinstitute.org]

Dr. Patrick J. Fox, is Professor of Medical Sociology and Health Policy, Department of Social and Behavioral Sciences and Co-Director, Institute for Health & Aging at the University of California, San Francisco. He received his Master of Social Welfare from the University of California, Berkeley and his Doctor of Philosophy in Sociology from the University of California, San Francisco where he was also a Pew Health Policy Scholar. He is the recipient of the UCSF School of Nursing's Helen Nahm Award for outstanding research contributions. He has also been elected as a Fellow of the Gerontological Society of America. Dr. Fox's interests include the sociology of aging, long-term care, health services research, health policy, Alzheimer's disease, economic costs of illness, and health promotion. He has written numerous reports and articles on the delivery of community-based long-term care, evaluations of health and long-term care services, the history of Alzheimer's disease, the emergence of the Alzheimer's disease social movement, and the economic costs of Alzheimer's disease.

[www.ucsf.edu and sbs.ucsf.edu/iha/]

Sharon Mercer is a writer and oral historian. For more than twenty years, she has worked with foundations, municipalities, schools, universities and corporations across North America. Mercer is the founder and president of Callisto, a company that specializes in oral and written histories. Callisto is based in Stinson Beach, California.

[www.callistoltd.com]